PRAISE FOR THIS BOOK

"Nutrition is fundamental to our brain health. Time after time, the research and clinical outcomes prove that our dietary choices have a profound effect on our function. In *How to Feed a Brain*, Cavin uses his own personal experience as an example and creates an easy-to-implement road map of nutritional changes to support your brain function and repair. The concepts he discusses are supported by a growing body of research evidence. This book is a welcome tool for people with neurological conditions and anyone who wants to optimize their brain performance."

- **Dr. Mark Hyman, MD,** *ten-time #1* New York Times *bestselling author, internationally-recognized leader, speaker, educator, and advocate in his field; Director of the Cleveland Clinic Center for Functional Medicine; Founder and Medical Director of The UltraWellness Center*

"*How to Feed a Brain* will change your life. ... If you have a brain injury or brain disease, or simply want to avoid early memory loss, and want to have a step-by-step guide for making tube feeds, soups, stews and or meals that will nourish and repair your brain, this book is for you."

- **Dr. Terry Wahls M.D.**, *researcher, speaker, and author of* The Wahls Protocol: A Radical New Way to Treat All Chronic Autoimmune Conditions Using Paleo Principles

"Ten years ago most health professionals would have scoffed at the notion that what we eat, how we sleep, and how we move, could have profound impacts on our health in general, and our brain health in particular. Fortunately, this outdated paradigm is shifting, and *How To Feed A Brain* will be a key piece of this change."

- **Robb Wolf**, *former research biochemist and two-time* New York Times/Wall Street Journal *Best-Selling Author of* The Paleo Solution *and* Wired To Eat

"This book is going to help many readers. I applaud Cavin for doing so much research and citing so much good scientific literature to ensure that his ideas are scientifically sound and accurate. I think it is remarkable that he has used his own traumatic experience to learn how to help himself as well as others. This practical nutritional advice is a welcome addition to the field. The information is presented in such a logical, clear fashion that it should be a resource book for anyone trying to optimize their brain health with improved nutrition."

- **Dr. Bonnie Kaplan Ph.D.**, *Emeritus Professor of Medicine at the University of Calgary*

"[T]he book [is] packed with sound, detailed information, [and] it provides precise how-tos and in-depth prescriptions for reclaiming your health and your brain. It is not only a valuable resource for those trying to recover from a brain injury, but a great guide for anyone who is looking to improve and optimize their brain's functioning. ... Cavin presents complicated science and essential information in an easy to understand and approachable manner. ... If you're dealing with any kind of brain injury and trying to regain your footing and restore some balance to your life, read this book."

- **Dr. Alessandra Wall, Ph.D.**, *Founder of Life in Focus Coaching, Licensed Clinical Psychologist*

"How to Feed a Brain is a veritable treasure trove of cutting edge nutritional wisdom and research, readily accessible and immediately applicable. ... I predict this book will be a lifesaver for many. ... I am a 30-year practicing physical therapist...and have worked with hundreds of TBI patients. ... I cannot wait to share this powerful and paradigm-shifting work with colleagues and peers and anyone who is ready for the simple truth that our nutrition is the fuel for bodies and brains and choosing the right nutrition for target cells is THE medicine for the future."

- **Dr. Melanie R Carlone, DPT, MS, RYT**

"Cavin's remarkable journey of recovery from a severe and traumatic brain injury to an active and fulfilling life serves as the backdrop for the key nutrition and lifestyle information and advice for optimal brain health detailed in *[How to]* Feed a Brain. The information on how an anti-inflammatory diet is linked to healing and maintaining neurological function is backed with clear and succinct explanations and scientific evidence. Additionally, Cavin incorporates practical guidance and recipes that cover the gamut from gastric feedings to eating a nutrient-rich diet. Reading *[How to] Feed a Brain* will educate and benefit not only those recovering from a traumatic brain injury, but anyone facing cognitive decline or attention issues, as well as looking to achieve and maintain maximum brain health and functioning.

- **Andrea Nakayama**, *Functional Nutritionist, Owner & Founder of Functional Nutrition Alliance*

"For anyone recovering from brain injury, Cavin Balaster's book *How to Feed a Brain is* the critical link between theory and application. ... Cavin's book fills the gap between what we understand about the importance of nutrition in brain recovery, and what that nutrition should look like. His recommendations are evidence-informed and practical. And given the reality that many patients with acute brain injury are reliant on tube feeds for some time, his advice on gastric feedings is especially helpful. I am unaware of any other publication that describes in such detail how nutritious whole foods can be reformulated as whole food tube feeds."

- **Venu R. Julapalli, M.D.**, *Founder, Integral Gastroenterology Center, P.A. Co-Founder, Conscious Medicine*

"Cavin has managed to take nutrition -- one of the many facets needed to calm the body and help healing -- and describe it as a large concept, then break it into pieces that are easy to understand and digest (pun intended). His book offers a large volume of nutritional information and guidelines for the healing layperson, and even has sections for people needing gastric tubes. ... When I met Cavin, he had me in tears as he described his heartfelt firsthand knowledge of what a patient has to go through to survive. He has found his calling in life."

- **Deborah Zelinsky, O.D.**, *an optometrist who researches brain function, Mind-Eye Connection, Northbrook, IL*

"Cavin Balaster's new book, *How to Feed a Brain*, is a must-read for anyone seeking optimal brain health. It is especially vital for those who've experienced traumatic brain injury, or who care for a TBI survivor. For athletes, soldiers, and others at risk of concussion, it offers protective nutritional strategies to minimize brain injury and accelerate recovery."

- **Randy Hartnell**, *President & CEO Vital Choice Wild Seafood & Organics*

"How to Feed A Brain is an excellent resource for patients, families, and clinicians on the journey towards better brain health. ... The information is well researched and complex topics such as neurophysiology and inflammation are explained in a way that any reader will understand. The standard of care for brain injuries is shifting and this book is a great catalyst to propel that shift."
    - **Dr. Kelsey Brenner DC, DACNB, FABBIR,** *Co-Owner*
        South Florida Integrative Health

"What an amazing tale of a brain's journey on its path to recovery! A musician's brain that had once effortlessly directed the complex movements of strumming guitar strings, through an unfortunate free-fall accident, lost its ability to initiate the simplest of daily essential movements. Not only did Cavin beat all odds in becoming self-sufficient by way of multi-disciplinary, functional-based therapies; he learned how to maximize his brain's potential by thoughtful nourishment. ... This book is a must-read for anyone wanting to supply their or their loved one's brain with building blocks for a solid foundation in optimal brain health. It is a must-have tool for any clinician to share with patients in need."
    -**Jesús L. Barrios, OD,** *Barrios Vision*

"Cavin Balaster has an extreme passion for improving the current standards of neurorehabilitation and brain optimization for all individuals. Not only does he offer insight into the complexity of the neuro-immunological and inflammatory cascade that occurs in traumatic brain injury, but he has lived it, researched it, and spent thousands of hours taking this knowledge and putting together *How to Feed a Brain*. It is a must read for anyone who is looking to improve their overall brain health."
    - **Dr. Jeremy Schmoe DC, DACNB, FABBIR**, *Owner of Minnesota Functional Neurology (mnfunctionalneurology.com)*

"Cavin Balaster has accomplished something important in the field of nutrition and self-healing that few authors have been able to do, made even more remarkable by his own experience with traumatic brain injury. By tapping into the latest research, combined with universal principles of health, Cavin has made his book about recovery from traumatic brain injury an exceptional source of information and inspiration for anyone."
    -**Reed Davis,** *Founder of Functional Diagnostic Nutrition Certification*

HOW TO
FEED A BRAIN

NUTRITION FOR OPTIMAL
BRAIN FUNCTION AND REPAIR

CAVIN BALASTER

Inquiries should be addressed to the Publisher:

Feed A Brain LLC

2407 S. Congress Ave.

Ste. E #775

Austin, TX 78704

ISBN: 978-0-9995002-1-7

Printed in the United States of America

BOOK DESIGN BY DANIELLE ACEE, ELISABETH A. WILSON, & CAVIN BALASTER

COVER DESIGNS BY ANUP KUMAR RAY & CAVIN BALASTER

HANDOUT DESIGN BY CHRISTA KNOX & CAVIN BALASTER

ILLUSTRATIONS BY RANDI SOUTHARD

EDITED BY ELISABETH A. WILSON

In 2012, Ryan Concannon sustained a severe traumatic brain injury and was comatose for months. During this time, he was to be fed the processed liquid formula commonly given to patients who are unable to eat orally. After learning of the awful ingredients in almost all feeding formulas, Ryan's mother, Patty, and his sister, Megan, fought to get Ryan a real food diet. They were successful, and have been great motivators in the writing of this book. I dedicate this guide to my friends, Patty, Megan, and Ryan Concannon. May this book influence the change in hospital nutrition that we work toward.

DISCLAIMERS

COPYRIGHT PERMISSION

HOW TO SUPPORT THIS WORK

This work is almost entirely independent of outside financial influence, which allows for more clear and accurate information. This also means that many unpaid hours from myself and several editors/reviewers went into its creation and refinement after years of careful research, sleepless nights, early mornings, referencing, reviewing, and editing. Please respect the effort, the protections, copyrights, and trademarks.

This book contains affiliate links which allow us to receive a percentage of any product or service you purchase using those links. If you are purchasing using our affiliate link, you will not pay a different price for the products and services, but your purchase helps support our ongoing work. Thanks for your support!

If you'd like to make a contribution to support this work and ongoing projects like it, I would be very grateful. Visit http://feedabrain.com/support or send your contribution directly via www.PayPal.com to:
donate@feedabrain.com.

TRADEMARK NOTICE

The term Feed a Brain is a trademark of Feed a Brain LLC. Whenever the term Feed a Brain is used in this book or associated handouts, it is referring to Feed a Brain™. For practitioners, a small fee may be paid to license the charts, handouts, and guides in this book for informational use with patients or the public. Visit feedabrain.com/license for more details.

TABLE OF CONTENTS

FOREWORD
By Dr. Datis Kharrazian DHSc, DC, MS

You are your brain. The health of your brain dictates everything about you. How you perceive life, your personality, your emotional health, and so on. A brain that has lost its function translates into lost passion and motivation, loss of enjoyment of things once loved, reduced function at work, hobbies, and as a contributing partner in relationships. An unhealthy brain can lead to depression, loneliness and isolation.

Many American habits are disastrous for the brain, and even more so for the injured brain. Childhood brain development disorders, dementia, mood disorders, and other brain-based disorders are at an all-time high as a result. Americans have normalized diets high in sugars and starchy carbohydrates, gluten, cheap fried foods, and other inflammatory foods. Westerners overeat, crash from skipping meals, boost energy with sugar and caffeine, then wonder why they can't function or sleep well. High stress and sedentary living round out the perfect recipe for brain degeneration.

Unlike the body's immune system, the brain's immune system does not have an off switch. Brain inflammation can continue unchecked for years, even decades, without anti-inflammatory and nutritional intervention.

This book is not the kind of information you will find in the standard health care model. Most brain injury patients are unlikely to receive quality nutritional advice from their health care provider. I have always found this curious considering how deeply sensitive the brain is to everything we eat, and how eagerly it responds to proper care and feeding. We also have much high-quality published research showing us what constitutes good brain nutrition.

So why aren't doctors doing more for brain injured patients?

Brain care is not part of the common care paradigm in neither conventional nor alternative medicine. Both branches are "neck-down" focused, despite the brain's high vulnerability to poor diet and chronic stress. Practitioners do not know how to recognize or manage the early stages of brain degeneration until it has progressed to a pathology past the point of return (Alzheimer's, Parkinson's, etc.) The cues of early brain degeneration can be subtle — words getting stuck on the tip of your tongue, worsened balance, diminishing sense of smell, or slowness of thinking and movement. Do not depend on the current health care model or wait until you have advanced symptoms before taking action. No one will ever care about your brain as much as you.

Cavin has used his journey recovering from a serious brain injury to share the tools and strategies that not only can help brain injury survivors, but likewise help anyone who wants the best performance from their brain. Being given less than a 10% chance of survival after his injury, Cavin was unable to eat, walk, or talk for months and was in a severe brain fog until he found functional medicine and functional neurology. As he slowly regained his health with a whole foods diet adapted for tube feeding, his clarity returned and he began to study why nutrition played such a large role in his brain recovery. Many of these strategies were learned through educational courses I teach to health care practitioners and have since published in *Why Isn't My Brain Working?* Cavin has become a spokesperson, author, and advocate not only for brain injury survivors and their loved ones, but also for those looking for better brain health. His enthusiasm has been a welcome boon to these fields.

Whether you are a brain injury survivor, have a loved one with a neurodegenerative disease, or you are simply looking to optimize your brain function, Cavin's book will teach you how to take care of your brain in the way it desires—and deserves.

- Datis Kharrazian, DHSc, DC, MS, MNeuroSci, FAACP, DACBN, DABCN, DIBAK, CNS
Author of *Why Isn't My Brain Working? A Revolutionary Understanding of Brain Decline and Effective Strategies to Recover Your Brain's Health*

ACKNOWLEDGMENTS & APPRECIATION

The words that it would take to adequately express the appreciation I have for the long list of those who have contributed to the rekindling of my life would be enough to fill these pages at least ten times over! And that tome of appreciation would not even have room to make mention of the beautiful and brilliant souls and capable practitioners who have not only contributed to the knowledge that was implemented to optimize my recovery but who have also contributed to the richness of my new life.

This section of the book only scratches the surface of my appreciation. If you have touched my life in a positive way, especially since May 2011, I trust that you know who you are, and that you know that I appreciate you.

I first want to acknowledge that I would not be alive to create this work if not for those who salvaged the physical hardware of my brain and body after a brain injury left me in a coma with less than a 10% chance of recovery. Their actions have literally saved my **life** and have given me the physical ability to write. I also would like to acknowledge those who have shared the **love** that kept me motivated through the hardest and most painful times that I have ever experienced… those who have given me the opportunity to reclaim its meaning. Additionally, I would like to acknowledge the many professionals who have shared their expertise and **light**… those who have helped to illuminate the landscape of my recovery and brain optimization so that I am able to navigate this rocky terrain and to help others to do the same. It excites me beyond comprehension that I am now able to share with the world some of what I have learned from what they illuminated for me!

Life:

Let's begin with those who have literally saved my life. First, I acknowledge my friends who sent for help after my fall, including Jon and Chloe Tronics, Pudge, Nate (RIP), Zak, Talon, and especially Seattle Steve. I am so glad to still be among most of you since the events of that night left little hope. I then want to thank the EMTs who brought me from the scene of my severe traumatic brain injury, to the hospital where emergency medicine and critical care doctors tended to my condition in 2011. Even though I never consciously met any of these people, I know that they and other emergency care professionals have saved countless lives, and they are rarely ever given the opportunity to even hear the voices of the lives they save. I have gone through my medical records where the name of the head physician who was in charge of saving my life appears at least a hundred times, and I believe that I would be dead - very dead - if not for the expertise and leadership of Dr. Scott D. Weingart MD. My thanks, gratitude, and appreciation for the work he and his team have done, and continue to do, is unquantifiable.

I would also like to express my appreciation for every nurse, therapist, and doctor who helped to nurture my recovery after waking from both my first and second coma. While I have little to no memory of those who helped me in the early stages, I want to especially thank (in no particular order) Alicia Multari Figon, Gina Abersante, Joy Romanovich, Nehal Patel, Peter Wu, Mara, Paulina, Josephina (Pinky), Mandy, Julie, Nadia, Hannah Kaplan, Yuwell, Holly, Sibhan, Melissa, Dr. Brian Greenwaldt, Dr. Tamar Kotz, and especially Dr. Brett Miles MD, who performed the throat surgery that gave me my voice back. I would also like to acknowledge Elmhurst Hospital Center in Queens, and Mount Sinai's Klingenstein Clinical Center in Manhattan, New York - the venues in which these professionals performed the heroic acts that brought me back to the point where I was medically stable and on my way towards recovery. My life would have looked very different if it weren't for the joint efforts of all of these professionals and so many more of whom I am not even aware or who my memory has not retained or remembered the importance of. Again, I am sure that there are many notable professionals who I have failed to mention, but my appreciation for them all is strong.

When it came to the direction of the quality of the medical care that I received, the tenacity, protection, and advocacy of my amazingly strong mother was likely the most important factor that determined my recovery. She traveled halfway across the country and was by my side to hold my comatose hand within hours. She advocated for my care and stuck by my side until I was able to carry my own again, and I cannot adequately express how grateful I am for everything that she has done. I am also eternally appreciative for the graciousness of her and her her fiance, John, for welcoming me into their home after my five-month hospitalization. I would also like to express my gratitude for my brother for pushing me to excel, and for my father, who always believed in me and supported my recovery and growth spiritually, financially, lovingly, and with encouragement.

Love:

While I would not be alive if not for the imperative attention of the doctors, nurses, and therapists who repaired the physical hardware of my brain and body, and my recovery would have been very different if not for the advocacy of my mother, I know that their work, as well as my mother's strength, was facilitated and enhanced by the community that showed their support. By reaching out, helping with the financial burden, or by even actually showing up, the community's love elevated my numerous healers' abilities to heal me, while without a doubt, also giving me a subconscious incentive to heal myself.

Some of those who especially showed their support from afar include my amazing family: my aunts: Tina, Helen, Lori, and Carol (who each sent a card several times a month while I was in the hospital), the Bernardo family, Chaplin Fullmer, the Long family, Howard Begor, Aunt Shirley and Uncle Paul, Bill Snavely, Rex, Marlene, and Taylor Welden, Lauri, Bernie and Jim Huey, Cousin Gina, Sean Winters, Webbjamin Ben, Scott Hendry, Sara Kinney, Naomi Waibel, Sarafina, Sarah and Laura Dembosky, Spencer and Sean Foreman, Morgan and Dallas Tuttle, Hugh Gordon, the Faurots, Tristan Waters, Joti Poirier, Jenn Strano, Geoff Rickly, Alex Saavedra, Ed Zipco, Andrew Sturgess, Heather Long, Britt Madden, Emilee Wallace, Sherill Kumbarji, Jenna Hodges, Emily Keane, David Butler, Elise Butler, Laurel Butler, Marissa Mickelberg, Adrien Segal, Tony Long, Tovah France, Jenn Strano, Orion Bridgehouse, Leah and Daniel Lakstins, Addy Fox, Sandi Calistro, Daniel Grits, Ali Zullo, Andrew Ritter, Tim Cleary, Anton Glamb, Fiona Bond, Justin Cline, Lauren Goodman, Lauren Byers, Angie Sullivan, Ali Dedianko, Thais Queiroz, Sam Franklin, Ariel Goldstein, Matt and Ashley

Gerathy, Audrey Sykes, Lina Suran, Karla Rodriguez, The Majestic Great Horned Owl (I'll be staying classy just for you), John Paget, Kim Gerards, and especially my strong and effective "other mother," Anna McDermott, who was unable to be there for us physically, but who was an enormous support from afar. These people (and one majestic owl) were a consistent reminder of those who cared about my preservation and growth, and their tokens of appreciation made more of a difference than they will ever truly know.

The psychology associated with such a devastating loss was not only softened by those who sent their love, support, and well wishes from afar, but especially by those who actually came to my hospital room to play cards with the disabled, voiceless, and sometimes angry man that I was. I especially would like to acknowledge and express my immense appreciation for Lyndsay, Jenn, Booz, Station, Zak, Kate, Jami, Lo, Tiana, Debbie W, Crystal, Rhana, Rebecca, Bones, Pudge, Ben Boi Boi, Jesse P, Atira, Shin K, Lauren Pratt, Trish, Tania Nadine, Lindsey Unger, Amanda Castello, Sam Distefano, Benj, Jessie P, Stina Nelson, Robert Viscuzi, Marisa Hast, Danny Lioneyes, Andrew Sturges, Shane, Tobin, Eddie, Jeremy Yocum, Tony Long, Catt, Aunt Barbara, my Beautiful Queen Aunt Debbie, Jason Cousins, Jaime Costigan, and the one and only Johnny Alexander. You guys rock, and I love each and every one of you.

Light:
In the reclamation of my brain's abilities after my several month hospitalization, I would like to make mention of, and to show my appreciation for some of those who played a large role in the coaching and direction of many different aspects of my recovery. Some of these people include Emily Brown Dunlap, Maggie Susong, Julie Holmsley, Robert Nurisio, Dr. Denise Smith, Dara Allen, Julio, Nani Bacon, Melissa Christopher Afflerbach, Mindy Raymond Benson, Meghan McCracken, Gabriel Martins, Pam Killeen, Dara Allen, Julie Stoots, Dr. Barbara Harris, Barker Franklin Keith, Kathryn Hayes, and Dr. Thomas Culleton. I would also like to thank my Aunt Debbie again, this time for steering me and my mother towards functional medicine, functional neurology, and neuro optometry. The trajectory of my life, and subsequently the lives of many others, would have looked very different had my exposure to these modalities not been illuminated for me.

As you will read in the upcoming pages of this book, at one point I was introduced to a nutritional practice, and it was after beginning this protocol that I began to regain clarity. Dr. Thomas Culleton DC, DACNB was the practitioner who showed me how the brain and the gut are very tightly related, and I am forever appreciative to have had him amongst my healing team. While working with Dr. Culleton, I realized that many of the answers to my healing were not practiced in the standard medical model. It was through Dr. Culleton's direction, graciousness, patience, and care that I learned how to regain the clarity I needed to research everything that I could to optimize my recovery.

While this may seem a little obvious and silly today, I'd also like to acknowledge the powerful resource that is the Internet, which gave me an opportunity to read (what little I could tolerate), to watch videos, and to listen to podcasts and recordings of important information that would ultimately be paramount to my healing. The Internet also gave me the opportunity to then reach out to practitioners across the globe, some of whom contributed their time and attention to my questions and requests and who helped me further. The most notable practitioner who responded in support of my contact has to be Dr. Alex Vasquez DO, ND, DC, who you will read about further in this book.

What you will not read in the body of this book is the story of my experience when I physically met Dr. Vasquez, so I will tell you about it here. In 2013, I reached out to Dr. Vasquez to introduce myself and to thank him for the online resources that he makes available. The timing was such that he invited me to attend the International Conference on Human Nutrition and Functional Medicine (ICHNFM), noting that there would be an entire day dedicated to the brain. This would be the first of many medical conferences that I would attend. I am so honored to have been given the opportunity to get on a plane for the first time after my injury to attend this medical conference with hundreds of practitioners and students.

While at the conference, on the day that was dedicated to the brain, Dr. Vasquez asked me what the most effective therapy was that I did for my brain after my injury. I responded by saying, "Honestly… healing my gut was what made all of the other therapies effective." We began to talk about the gut-brain axis (which you will read more about), and at one point, Dr.

Vasquez said, "Ya know... We need you on stage." Then, looking at his watch he asked, "How do you feel about being on stage in about 20 minutes?"

The next thing I knew, I was giving an impromptu presentation to a hall filled with hundreds of medical students and practitioners. After giving a short synopsis of my story and illustrating why nutrition is so paramount to brain health, Dr. Vasquez said a few words about the importance of a patient perspective and the crowd began clapping. As I looked over the audience of practitioners and students who would make up much of the future of medicine, I realized that I could make a difference in neurorehabilitation, and my path began to crystallize.

Since attending this conference, I have continued to stay in touch with Dr. Vasquez, and I have an enormous amount of appreciation and respect not only for the loads that he manages to accomplish, but more importantly, for the quality and integrity of his work. His heart is absolutely in the right place and he ensures that his work is held to the highest standards of science, clinical applicability, ethics, social effect, and influence. I am inexplicably appreciative of Dr. V, and I am so honored to call him a mentor.

I also met many very important people at this conference, starting with Dr. David Haase, who first introduced me to the framework of story, soup, skill, and spark, Deanna Minnich, who taught me about phytonutrients, Elaine Marshall (Fawcett), who illustrated for me the importance of the work I was soon to do (and who would eventually facilitate in this book's influence), and especially Andrea Nakayama, a functional nutritionist who you will read more about in this book. Andrea would eventually take me on to her team where I would prepare course materials for her online functional nutrition training, exposing me to so much more that would prepare me to become who I would need to be in order to accomplish what I have since this injury. I have so much appreciation not only for the opportunities that she has provided, but for everything that she is, the work that she does, and the light that she radiates. You can learn more about Andrea and her practitioner training at feedabrain.com/hnl.

Following this conference, I launched a crowdfunding campaign to raise money to write a book, which would transform into what you are now holding. This campaign was only successful because of the support of so many, including Laurel Butler and Ewen Wright, who worked with me to create the video for the campaign. I want to again thank the entire Butler family, especially to Laurel's little sister, Elise, and their amazing father, David Butler. Not only did both Elise and David donate to help me as soon as they heard that I was in the hospital with a brain injury, but they both also contributed to my Kickstarter campaign. What's more, their help in promoting the video made a huge difference in spreading the word and in ensuring the success of the campaign. Some of the more notable financial backers of this book include the VisionHelp Group, Ellen C. Burgess, Devin Doyle, David Butler, Jesús L. Barrios, OD, Kelly Meazell, Eli Fries, Uncle Rob, Aunt Barbara, my mama, my papa, Billy Jo Bailey, Donna Moore, Sherill, Lucas Steuber, Andrew Ritter, Kara Heying, and again... My Beautiful Queen Aunt Debbie! My appreciation for these, and the more than 250 other backers of the book is absolutely enormous, as this book may have not been possible without them.

Since the ICHNFM conference and subsequent crowdfunding, a dear friend stepped in to help me to live into the path that my life has been aimed towards. The enormous appreciation that I have for Alek Hess cannot be overstated, as his collaboration, smarts, and hard work towards these projects has been far above and beyond. Alek helped to provide me with an online platform to launch my work in an attractive way, he built the launch pad and piloted the initial ascent of the Adventures in Brain Injury Podcast, he has assisted in creating and curating much of the content that I produce, and he has played a keystone role in creating what has led to further opportunities for me to help people to navigate their brain recovery or to optimize their brain function. I could not have done this without him, and my gratitude and appreciation for Alek Hess is tremendous.

Next... I can hardly express the delight that I have in taking this opportunity to recognize my magnificent co-host, Michelle Malmberg, for joining the adventures. This podcast has become one of the most powerful aspects of my life and I am honored to share the virtual stage with her. The personable energy, thoughtful questions, and playful interview style that she brings to the show speaks the exact tone that I had envisioned. Not to mention that Michelle and I get to interview the smartest and most inspirational people that we've ever even heard of, about tools that can be utilized to optimize brain function and repair. We couldn't be more grateful for the opportunity, and I couldn't be more appreciative of the co-host who agreed to take the position (even if she is a smarty pants).

I would also like to thank the financial supporters of the Adventures in Brain Injury Podcast, who contribute as little as a buck per episode but whose contributions help us to cover the cost of producing the show. I'd especially like to again give my thanks and appreciation to Dr. Mary Van Hoy (Gramma Flash Flash) as well as Sherill Kumbarji and Katharine Hess for their contributions to our Patreon page.

I am also eternally grateful for the social programs that have made my recovery possible and I would like to thank Anne Forrest, Amy Zelmer, Greg Ayotte, Paul Bosworth, and others who advocate for policy that helps those with brain injury, brain disease, and other chronic conditions in which therapy is helpful. I would also like to show my appreciation and support for the American Congress of Rehabilitation Medicine (ACRM), the Brain Injury Research Center at Mount Sinai, the Model Systems Knowledge Translation Center (MSKTC), the Patient-Centered Outcomes Research Institute (PCORI), the National Institute on Disability, Independent Living, and Rehabilitation Research (NIDILRR), the Texas Department of Assistive and Rehabilitative Services (DARS), the International Association of Functional Neurology and Rehabilitation (IAFNR), the Carrick Institute, and the Brain Injury Association of America (BIAA).

I am especially honored to express my appreciation for Charlene Crump, Chip Howe, Jim Parr, Dawn Winters, Bill Perkins, Anne Marie, Cliff, Tanner, and the rest of the team at the Mary Lee Foundation in Austin, Texas. The creation and work of this Foundation and the core team that turns its wheels has transitioned hundreds of brain injury survivors towards a better life and its assistance in doing so has been an invaluable resource to me and to so many others in the local brain injury community. I would also like to make mention of Bonnie Lastor for her help in steering me in their direction. In addition, I'd like to make mention of Zane, Glenn, Sam, Troy, and especially Stacey for putting up with and for supporting me through my apparent workaholism in the writing of this book.

I am also so grateful to have the honor to acknowledge the many who have made this work possible, either by teaching me, by opening doors for me, or both. Dr. Terry Wahls, MD has been the strongest, most brilliant, and supportive force that has made this book such a powerful possibility, and my appreciation for who she is, the work she has done, and the work she continues to do, cannot be understated. Not only has Dr. Wahls helped hundreds of thousands to reclaim their lives after receiving the diagnosis of a debilitating condition of Multiple Sclerosis, but her work has been a massive aspect to my recovery, and what it means to Feed a Brain. Without her support, notoriety, and the connections that she has shared, this book would not be possible. I would again like to thank Andrea Nakayama for arranging an introduction with Dr. Wahls, and Diane V. Capaldi for being the miracle boss lady that she is and for being such a strong support and friend.

I would also like to express my gratitude for the guidance and contributions of Laura Schoenfeld, MPH, RD, Jeremy Lampel, MS, RD, CDE, Kathryn Hayes CCC-SLP, Katy Haldiman RN, Dr. Richard Wurtman, Dr. Richard Feinman, and again, Dr. Alex Vasquez DC, ND, DO, FACN and Dr. Terry Wahls MD. Some other notable names who have been an enormous help in some shape or form, whether they know it or not, include (list in no particular order): Dr. Datis Kharrazian, Dr. Vilayanur Ramachandran, Dr. David Perlmutter, Dr. Lauren Noel, John Medina, Jessica Flanigan, Dr. Jim LaValle, Prof. Daphne Koller, Prof. Peggy Mason, Prof. Idan Segev, Linus Pauling, Michele Vincenzo Malacarne, Donald Hebb, Camillo Golgi, Santiago Ramón y Cajal, Elizabeth Gould, Fred H. Gage, Viktor Frankl, Jean Dominique Bauby, Kyle Maynard, Martin Pistorius, Dr. Loren Cordain, Chris Kresser, Dr. Richard Feinman, Sean Croxton, Nora Gedgaudas, Dr. Kelly Brogan, Dr. Alessandra Wall, Dr. Leonard Press, Dr. Curtis Baxtrom, Dr. Charles Shidlofsky, Dr. Robert Sanet, Dr. Lynn Hellerstein, Jenny Garbus, Dr. Deborah Zelinsky, the Neuro Optometric Rehabilitation Association (NORA), Dr. Babak Kateb, Dr. Norman Doidge, Kevin Pearce, Marianna Sackler, Katherine and Kevin Valias, Dr. Craig Reese, Leila Noone, Will and Susan Revak, Krystal Williams, Adrian Giannotta, Dr. Bonnie Kaplan, Dr. Ted Carrick, Tricia Carrick, Lindsey Dumm, Ginger, Amy, Chris Masterjohn, Brian Richards, Amazing Grace, Joe Bones, Dr. Corinne Scalzitti, Steve Wright, Sage Francis, Ian Cooke, Tom Waits, Pete Bernhard, Charles Holmes, Megan Moore, Elisabeth Walter, Dr. Dan Pardi, Diana Lane, Sarah and Laura Dembosky (again and again), Stephanie Smith, Marco Santori, Rick Hamilton, Emily Hollis, Gregory Nardello, Rob Abrams, Adam Greenberg, Benj, Kathy Karlo, Zoe Hayes, Ali Miner, Will Stewart, Raoul, Elroy, Randi Southard, Clare and Phil Gephart, Amy Moll, James Stephens, Dr. Dan Grangaard, Johnson's Backyard Garden, Susannah Cahalan, Montana Masback, Jordan Sorman, Zeem Rock, Pam Killeen, Alice Chan, Ali from 280, Adam Valez, Sharon Noah Workman, Emily Hollis, Ali Dedianko, Lindsey Cook, Peter Larkin, Josh Wright, Paul Peffer, James Felkner, Agent Red, Bryan Barksdale, Nick Gomez, Brian Williamson, Jimmy Moore, Dr. Richard Feinman, Ruth Willmore, Josh Kessler, John Hueber, Pamela Geismar, Tristan Truscott, David Gonzales, Vivian Kolenda, Ivan Nikolov, Jesse Elder, Josh B. Lee, Lina Marchman, Ali Miner, Nolan Aldridge, Makh Aten, Jim Keane, William Bird, Dan Pultz, Dr. David Okonkwo, Dr. Walt Schneider, Ali Patterson, Kate Edelman, Sharon Mundy, Jen Folker, Patty, Megan, and Ryan Concannon, Peter Magurean III, Chris Wilson and Bianca, Kelly Virginia Vinson, James Thorpe, Nick Wood, Mary Titus, Heather Long, Stephanie Ball, Dane and Dustin Rex, Wisam Alshaibi, Dr. Bruce Lipton, Dr. Jerome Lubbe, Michael Lievens, Crystal Benezra, Misty Willams, Shibani Subramanya, Randy Hartnell, Pam Killeen, James Boucher, Taylor Welden, Brian Takats, Chris Owens, Molly Richter, Natalie Myersick, Leslie Sisson, Scott Wirtalla, Jessica Chang, and especially Keith and Michelle Norris for their eternal support, graciousness, encouragement, patience, and their seemingly orchestrated nourishment of my growth and development. What they have built together with Paleo f(x) has been the catalyst to so much healing in the world, and I am honored to call them my friends.

I would also like to thank Dr. Jeremy Schmoe for introducing me to many important practitioners and influencers who could further my mission; Carriann Terzini for her encouragement and belief and for working along my side to influence the lives who need us the most; and Dr. Josh Flowers, Dr. Manuel Nuñez, Dr. Scharlene Gaudet, and the rest of the team at Revive Treatment Centers, not only for being the coolest team of functional neurologists I know, but also for being such a collaborative team towards their patients' wellbeing.

When it comes to the physical manifestation of this book, I would like to acknowledge and to show my appreciation to Christa Knox for putting so much work into the design of the original handout drafts; Randi Southard for doing much of the sketches, diagrams, and artwork; Danielle Acee, for being the midwife to the birth of this book; and especially to Elisabeth A. Wilson, JD, OT who brought her skills, expertise, and attention to detail to the editing, reference checking, formatting, and design process of this book. Her work guided this book to the place where it needed to be to make a powerful impact. She also lent her expertise to the creation of FeedaBrain.com and the Feed a Brain Interview Series. I know that this could not have been done anywhere near to the degree that it was without her. My appreciation and eternal support for her is unwavering.

I'd like to again thank Randy Hartnell for introducing me to those who can make this book even more powerful; Zach Nasr for being aligned in all the right ways and for joining me in this mission; Lauren Andrews for her organizational magicianship; Ryan Withrow for being an enormous support, mentor, and friend, and for his love for metal and awesome communication; and Justin and Irina Litchfield for their mentorship, support, and encouragement for Feed a Brain. I would like to acknowledge and to show my appreciation for all of my reviewers, both professional and non, with a special mention of Melanie Carlone, Karen O'Loughlin, Allegheny Ray, and Daniel Burnham for the time and attention that was put towards fine tuning this book. Thank you guys for helping to hone my message to make sure that this book has the capability of being a strong force in the world.

Lastly, I feel it is important to take this opportunity to also acknowledge my appreciation for myself. There was a point where doing so was no easy task, but the demonstration of compassion, appreciation, and truthful expression with love that I am so fortunate to have received from many of the names mentioned have truly given me awareness. This awareness of my strengths and shortcomings and how I affect the lives around me has brought me the ability to know, love, and appreciate myself. In doing so, this work has become a true possibility. I feel blessed to pass on such a beautiful gift. By encouraging others to appreciate and to love themselves, we give them the tools to truly love and appreciate others and we sow the seeds that continue to heal the world. It all starts with loving yourself.

Thank you all for giving me the ability to acknowledge, appreciate, and to love myself.

Thank each and every one of you for your continued support to make this book shine bright enough to influence a positive change in healthcare.

Thank you for giving me the ability to speak my truth softly and powerfully. Thank you for showing me the authority in tranquility. Thank you for demonstrating the power in being cool, calm, and collected... the **Strength in Serenity**.

Thank you for showing unconditional support without a need for reciprocation. Thank you for illuminating a path for me to find and fulfill my purpose so that I may carry the torch and illuminate a path for others. Thank you for showing me your **Love and Light** so that I may become a carrier of love and light. And thank you all for helping me keep my playful nature. Thank you for keeping me true to the **Rock and Roll**... the playful connections that give us permission to indulge in the richness of life... the importance of pushing the edge... the enjoyment of life beyond the so called "rules." As you will read in these pages, and as a theme to this book, I believe that the healthiest thing we can do for our brains, bodies, and souls is to enjoy our lives and to do so sustainably.

Thank you for joining me on this adventure and the exciting adventures to come.

From the bottom of my heart and the deepest fissures of my brain, THANK YOU! THANK YOU! THANK YOU!

Strength and Serenity... Love and Light... Rock and Roll!

> - **Cavin Balaster**, CEO and Creator of FeedaBrain.com and AdventuresinBrainInjury.com, Speaker, Author, Coach, and Co-Host of the Adventures in Brain Injury Podcast

PREFACE

ABOUT ME

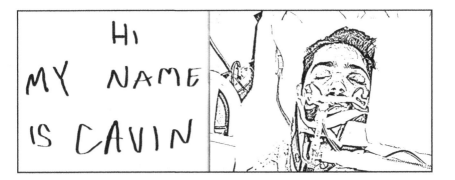

My name is Cavin Balaster.

In 2011, I fell 20 feet from a rooftop water tower scaffolding. My head struck a steel beam on the way down before crashing onto the concrete rooftop below. I was immediately rushed to the hospital and put on life support. While in a coma, an MRI revealed a severe diffuse axonal injury (DAI), which is one of the most devastating types of brain injury. Statistically, over 90 percent of patients with this injury never regain consciousness, and most of those who do will often remain in a persistent vegetative state.

I am very fortunate to be alive!

In the first few months following my accident, I endured two comas that lasted several weeks (one from the initial fall and one induced). I woke in a severe brain fog with significant memory loss, coordination issues with the left side of my body, and was unable to eat, walk, or talk for months.

I was breathing through a tube in my neck, receiving processed liquid hospital formula through a tube in my belly, and my left hand was completely flexed inward.

Prior to this event, I was a twenty-seven-year-old musician and entrepreneur making music and sharing it with the world. Whatever plans I had made for my life at that point came to a screeching halt when I found myself quite literally tied down to a hospital bed with no real guarantee that I would ever get up. I was a child once again—a twenty-seven-year-old child—completely dependent upon those around me.

Following the acute stages of my brain injury, I found myself in the most difficult of circumstances I could have imagined. My goals became a lot more simplistic. I was no longer asking myself when my next gig would be, but instead was asking myself when I could take a bite of real food again, when I could go outside, or when my inward flexed hand would return to a position where it could grip the neck of my guitar again. I needed to regain everyday faculties if I were ever to aim higher, and this realization stung. The life I had known was over and I had a long road ahead of me if I were to ever feel alive again.

Once my condition was stabilized, navigating the physical and emotional toll of my new circumstances was only a small part of what I would need to do to recover my brain function. There were times when I felt helpless and stuck, but I learned to use my frustration to motivate me to regain autonomy.

Despite the damage to my brain, I was able to recognize that wallowing in my misfortune would not bring me any closer to recovery. The injury I had sustained was like someone had hit the reset button on my cognitive and physical abilities, yet I was in a position where I could still observe myself learning and redeveloping. I would need to teach myself how to walk, talk, eat, balance, and handle a ball (or any object for that matter). I would also need to relearn how to think. I would need to relearn the actual process of learning so that I could teach my brain and body how to do all of the things that I had lost the ability to do, and I had lost so many of my abilities.

I did not know if I'd ever recover enough to lead a "normal life," but I vowed that if I did get better I would work to share the most effective tools that I found throughout my own recovery. The book you are holding is in line with that vow and you can find more on social media, guest appearances, the Adventures in Brain Injury Podcast, and on feedabrain.com.

WHY IS THIS BOOK ABOUT NUTRITION?

In the wake of my brain injury, I was lucky enough to be introduced to a particular eating and supplement regiment. Soon after implementing this nutritional practice, I began to regain clarity. I did not realize it at the time, but I had been in a fog since my injury. I had been in such a dense fog that I was not even aware that I was in a fog. How can one tell that it is raining when underwater?

I utilized my newfound clarity and found myself researching metabolism, neuro-metabolism, mechanisms of neuroplasticity, nutrients for synapto-genesis, and anything else I could do to optimize my recovery. I was soon contacting practitioners of many different specialties across the globe so that I could better understand everything I could about the plastic nature of the brain, or its ability to change and repair itself.

I was studying like my life depended on it…because it did.

If I were to come back from this, I knew I needed to understand how I could give my brain the best shot to recover, and there was clearly something to nutrition. I was committed to understanding how to feed my brain for optimal function and repair.

WHERE AM I NOW?

Today, six years after my injury, I write this with great appreciation, gratitude, and purpose as I have recovered beyond all expectations. I now drive, ride motorcycles, camp, play guitar, sing, swim, and practice martial arts! I even do back flips off of diving boards! With their expertise playing a monumental role in my recovery, I am now working with doctors, nutritionists, chiro-practors, neurologists, professors, dietitians, nurses, and therapists, (some of whom are also successful survivors) putting together resources that help guide others. My primary goal for sharing the information I've learned throughout my experience and work within many different medical communities, while beneficial for anyone, is helping survivors and their loved ones as they navigate the turbulent waters of recovery.

In the past few years, I have been invited to attend several medical conferences, the first of which being the International Conference on Human Nutrition and Functional Medicine, where I gave an impromptu speech to a room filled with hundreds of health practitioners and medical students. Subsequently, I have found myself on stage as the keynote speaker for several nationally recognized organizations such as the Neuro Optometric Rehabilitation Association and the Brain Injury Alliance of New Jersey. I have presented to hundreds of health practitioners as a guest speaker.

I have so much appreciation for the remarkable opportunities I have had, and continue to have, working with brilliant and talented individuals within health and medicine. Through my work with Andrea Nakayama's practitioner training, Holistic Nutrition Lab, I have had the opportunity to learn from cutting-edge MDs, DOs, naturopaths, and functional medicine practitioners daily. Andrea is a world-renowned functional nutritionist and health educator whose company provides what James Maskell of Functional Forums has called "the only scalable functional medicine training that exists." You can learn more about Holistic Nutrition Lab and their practitioner training at feedabrain.com/hnl.

Through the years which I have dedicated to the optimization of my brain function, and through the connections that I have established with amazing practitioners, I have put forth careful consideration of these topics. What you hold in your hands is the culmination, integration, and application of the nutritional building blocks that I have found to be most useful towards neurological health. I have also put much attention into streamlining and distilling these concepts so that more people can understand, and I am so honored to bring this book to you.

Let's begin!

Chapter 1
ABOUT THIS GUIDE

I wrote this book as a guide for those who are looking for brain support, whether for themselves, for their clients, or for their loved one. It may be due to a concussion, a more severe brain injury, a neurodegenerative process, or simply an interest in improving brain function. This book outlines what I learned from years of researching, corresponding, connecting, consulting, and working with many specialists within the medical community, functional practitioners, nutritionists, health educators, and other brain injury survivors. The most influential contributors with whom I consulted include Laura Schoenfeld, MPH, RD (Ancestralize Me), a Registered Dietitian with a Masters in Public Health Nutrition (MPH) and who has a strong background in functional medicine; Jeremy Lampel, MS, RD, CDE, a registered dietitian and certified diabetes educator with a Master's degree in nutritional science; Kathryn Hayes CCC-SLP, my speech language pathologist with over 30 years of experience with TBI patients ranging from comatose to more than 20 years post-injury; Katy Haldiman RN (The Paleo Nurse), a registered nurse and certified nutritional therapist with over 10 years of clinical experience; Dr. Alex Vasquez DC, ND, DO, FACN, an international lecturer and author of more than 120 professional/scientific articles and 20 books—including the two-volume *Textbook of Clinical Nutrition and Functional Medicine*; and Dr. Terry Wahls MD, a medical doctor who has overcome multiple sclerosis with diet and lifestyle. My hopes are to translate their expertise and to guide you as you learn how to feed your brain.

This book is not a promotion of the newest fad diet, nor was it written by a corporation capitalizing on unsubstantiated claims of brain enhancement. I am dedicated to bringing valuable information to those who want to improve their brain health and performance.

WHO IS THIS BOOK FOR?

Whether you are looking for a more successful recovery from injury, stroke, disease, pain relief, mood stability, or even a slimmer waistline, amazing things have been reported while practicing these principles. Focusing on a foundation of healthy digestion and nutrition, anyone interested in protecting or optimizing brain function can benefit greatly from implementing the practices in this book.

Not a day goes by that I don't hear about the significant, positive, and life-changing effects of conscious eating and healthy digestion. The right kind of nutrition really is one of the most important keys to sustainable health and function—be it headache and migraine relief, reduced dependence upon medications, mood stability, improved sleep, stroke recovery, brain injury, brain disease, or other neurological conditions.

In this guide, you'll learn about how food played a large role in my recovery from a near-fatal brain injury. You will hear the story of how Dr. Terry Wahls, a medical doctor diagnosed with progressive multiple sclerosis, used diet and lifestyle to thrive and overcome her reliance on a tilt-recline wheelchair. I am also going to tell you about how my friend and fellow co-host of the Adventures in Brain Injury Podcast, Michelle Malmberg, was given only a one percent chance of survival after a grand mal seizure left her with a Glasgow Coma Score (GCS) of only three (If a rock had a heartbeat it would have a GCS of three). Today, Michelle is alive, raising her child, enjoying her life, and even dancing again. She attributes much of her survival and recovered abilities to the power of the right nutrition. You can learn more about Michelle and the Adventures in Brain Injury Podcast on iTunes or at: adventuresinbraininjury.com/podcasts.

In 2015, the US National Institute of Mental Health (NIMH) estimated that 17.9% of American adults suffer from a diagnosable mental disorder in any given year.[1] We all want to protect our brains the best we can, and as you will see, many of the dietary practices outlined in this guide have been shown to prevent, reduce, and even reverse some of these disorders.

USING THIS GUIDE

While this information is valuable to anyone looking to improve their overall health and brain function, it may be most beneficial when used in a collaborative fashion with a partner, caretaker, therapist, nutritionist, health practitioner, or physician.

You will learn which whole foods and supplements act as building blocks for the brain. With recipes and guidelines of how to make many different dishes, using specific kinds of ingredients, you will learn how to make delicious smoothies, salads, soups, purees, and other dishes that will supply the brain with the nutrition it craves. You will also learn supplementation options and supplementation information, as well as solutions for nutritional enhancement, dietary restrictions, or possible food intolerances. For patients who are not able to eat conventionally and are receiving nutrition through a gastric tube, this book also explains how to supply better feeds, and advises you on how to work with your health care team in order to obtain nutritional support.

Optimally feeding the brain may require significant changes to diet and lifestyle, and in a hospital setting may require confrontation, requests, and finesse. After the initial dietary changes, you will see that optimally feeding the brain is a casual and enjoyable lifestyle.

This book is not about being dogmatic forever. This is about learning how your unique physiology reacts to the foods you eat and how those reactions affect your brain. With the powerful information you will derive, you will then have the freedom to make choices for better brain health. After all,

the healthiest thing we can do for our brains is to enjoy our life and to do so sustainably.

This book will give you the nutritional tools to do so.

Although this guide outlines practices that are very doable, they may be met with resistance. To effectively implement these guidelines, organization and effort are needed. To make things easier, we are also working to arrange for the availability of pre-made Feed a Brain approved meals that can be delivered to your door and then simply heated before eating.

Go to feedabrain.com/premade for more information.

SUPPLEMENTING THIS MEAL PLAN

What are supplements? Let's think about the word "supplement." The capsules, liquids, and powders that are often referred to as supplements are just that: nutrients to supplement, or to make up for a lack of, the nutrients that we obtain in the food we eat. Unless we are able to execute every aspect of this meal plan perfectly, we are likely going to be missing out on important nutrients that are tricky for us to obtain in our everyday diet. Unless, of course, we supplement strategically. Some nutrients are realistic for us to obtain from food in adequate amounts; however, others do not come so easy.

Supplementation Information

Throughout this book, you will find boxes like this to give supplementation options. To make things more organized for you, we have gathered and organized lists of suggested supplements at feedabrain.com/supplements.

Gastric Feed Information

If you or a loved one are unable to eat conventionally, there will be boxes like this throughout the book to explain what can be done when feeding via gastric feeds. If you are in need of this information, but do not have time to read through the entire book immediately, be sure to read Chapter 13: "Gastric Feeding Guidelines," near the end of the book. My experience has shown me how food can be extremely medicinal, so we are working with companies developing Feed a Brain approved meal replacement drinks and gastric feeds, which you can find at feedabrain.com/feeds. Additionally, high dose Omega-3s have been shown to be an extremely brain supportive addition after brain injury, but only when the oils are high quality and non-oxidized. For more information and some Feed a Brain approved, brain supportive oils go to feedabrain.com/omega.

Chapter 2
AN INTRODUCTION TO NUTRITION
AND THE BRAIN

WHAT IS THE BRAIN?

Shakespeare once wrote "the brain is the soul's fragile dwelling place," and fragile it is. The brain has the consistency of tofu, and brain injuries, strokes, or diseases often result in impairments. Our brains are made up of billions of nerve cells and fibers, networked by trillions of connections and synapses.[2] Yet, a hard skull, three layers of membrane, and a cushion of shock-absorbing fluid are all that protect the seat of our personality, emotions, actions, and abilities.[3]

Just a few decades ago, it was commonly believed that the nerve cells of the brain were unable to regenerate or repair themselves once the brain was fully developed—around the age of 25.[4, 5] This perception set clinical neurology on a trajectory for seeing the brain as a fixed organ throughout adulthood—a brain that is incapable of repairing itself after adult injury.[6]

Dr. Vilayanur S. Ramachandran, a Professor of the Graduate Program of Neurosciences at the University of California, San Diego, refers to this time as the "bronze age of neurology."[7] Thank goodness we've reached the age of reason. Today, we know that the brain is "plastic," or capable of change, and we're constantly improving our understanding of "neuroplasticity," and applying new strategies in the field of neurorehabilitation.

As outlined in Dr. Norman Doidge's book, *The Brain That Changes Itself,* "neuroplasticity is overthrowing the centuries-old notion that the human brain is immutable."[8] Featured in his book are the stories of those who regained the ability to speak after a stroke, whose aging brains became rejuvenated, and who were even blind and learned to see! In many ways, these stories mirror my own and are increasingly changing the way we understand neurorehabilitation.

In 1906, Santiago Ramon y Cajal shared the Nobel Peace Prize with Camillo Golgi for the discovery and imaging of the cellular structures of the nervous system.[9] Using the Golgi staining method, discovered by Camillo Golgi in 1873, the various elements that build the nervous system were revealed. What they were able to observe would later be called neurons, axons, and dendrites.[10] This information provided an understanding of the cellular structures involved in thought or action, which opened the door to countless future studies that support neuroplasticity.[11, 12]

We will talk more about brain plasticity and offer specific nutrients and supplements to support it, but to effectively grasp the fundamentals of brain plasticity, we first must understand the cellular structures within the brain.

What Makes up the Brain?

The primary functional cells of the nervous system are called neurons.[13] Neurons communicate with each other and allow us to do anything: think, move, see, eat, talk, swallow, smile, breathe, digest food, and absolutely everything else that we do. Neurons and their communications are vital to *every* function of life.[14]

A neuron is a living cell, but unlike other cells, neurons have several projections that come from their cell body. Let's think of these projections as phone lines. While many calls can be received (call waiting, conference calls, etc.), only one call can be sent out. The many projections that take in phone calls (or nerve pulses) are called dendrites, while the one projection that sends out and makes phone calls (or nerve pulses) is called the axon.[15]

The space where one neuron's axon and another neuron's dendrite meet is called the synapse: this is where communication between neurons occurs.[16]

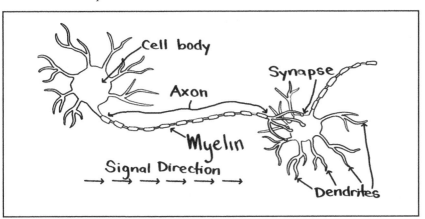

This neuronal communication is extremely efficient because of a fatty white substance called myelin. Myelin is a sheath that wraps around axons to increase the speed of a signal from one neuron to the next.[17] While this conductive sheath is used to efficiently transmit signals, in order for the signals to fire, energy is needed, and this energy ultimately comes from fuel.

How is the Brain Fueled?

Imagine a living cell as a vehicle with an engine that is always running. By weight, the majority of the fuel that the engine requires comes from the food we eat.

I'm going to say that again, because it was this understanding that was the most important lesson I made in my recovery (and my entire outlook on health):

Cells need the right fuel to function properly, and cellular fuel comes from food.[18]

The means by which the brain and body are fueled and repaired is known as metabolism, and metabolism is the most important way for us to support the cells in the brain.[19] When we eat food, drink water, and breathe air, biochemical reactions occur in the brain and body so that we can generate energy, grow, and heal. These biochemical reactions are collectively referred to as metabolism.[20] While we have little control over the quality of the air we breathe (beyond choosing not to smoke or purifying the air in our home), we have much more control over what we eat and drink. When we eat or drink, the process of breaking down what we've consumed into substances that can be used by the body is what we call digestion.[21]

11

THE GUT-BRAIN AXIS: DIGESTION & THE BRAIN

Did you know that the brain consumes more nutrients and oxygen than any other tissue in the body? Consisting of only about two percent of the weight of the human body, the brain uses at least 20 percent of the calories in the foods we consume! [22, 23, 24, 25, 26] As you can imagine, the nature of these calories is important to brain function and repair.

How does the Brain Repair?

Like every other part of the body, the brain heals and operates cell by cell. When cells malfunction or are damaged, eventually the organs made up of those damaged cells also malfunction. Whether it is the liver with cirrhosis, the intestinal lining with Crohn's Disease, the lungs with bronchitis, or the brain with a brain injury or neurodegenerative disease, the cell is what it all comes down to.

Neurons, which make up an estimated one-half of the cells of the brain, [27] give us the ability to do all the things we do. The other half of brain cells are special cells called glia cells, which consist of many different types.[28] Glia support the function of neurons so that they are in turn able to support the functions of the brain and body.[29] Borrowing an analogy from a mentor, Dr. Alex Vasquez, DC, ND, DO, FACN, let's think of neurons as plants, and the glia, or the cells that support neurons, like the soil that the plants are potted in. Much like how soil provides nutrients to a plant, glia provide nutrients to neurons so that they can grow, function, and repair.[30]

When the brain is diseased, damaged, or degenerating, we see damage to the neurons and the connections between them.[31, 32, 33] There are two very important aspects to building or rebuilding connections in the brain:

We need to supply the building blocks through nutrition, and we need to stimulate the growth of those neurons and the connections between them through targeted therapy.

I think of building new pathways in the brain like building a bridge. Doing therapy and putting in the work to stimulate the growth of neuronal pathways is like enlisting skilled workers to build a bridge. Providing the brain and body with the right nourishment is like supplying those workers with adequate tools and resources. We can have the best bridge architects, the most skillful designers, and the most seasoned workers, but

if we don't provide the right supplies and tools, the connections are not well built.

In other words, we can do the best and most targeted therapy, but without quality nutrition, the important connections within the brain will not be well established. Conversely, eating nutrient dense, brain building nutrition, but doing the wrong kind of therapy or no therapy at all is like having all the lumber that one would need to build a strong bridge, but no one (or only unskilled workers) to build it. In either scenario, a bridge, or new pathways in the brain, are not very well supported or established. Both skilled workers (targeted therapy) and the right building materials (brain building nutrition) are necessary.

There is so much to say surrounding what I consider to be the most beneficial therapies towards neurorehabilitation and performance optimization, including neuro-optometry and functional/chiropractic neurology (which you can learn more about at feedabrain.com/practitioners), but:

this book is all about how to supply the right building materials to the brain through nutrition.

As I learned how my actions and food choices could have a direct impact on my brain, I began to *eat my way* to regained clarity and was able to escape my brain fog, and I'm not alone. Many other survivors with whom I've worked and spoken have reported similar results.

There is an ancient and deep connection between the body's digestion and nervous system, dating back to the very first organisms. Among other abilities such as reproduction, all known types of organisms can carry out some kind of metabolic reactions (digestion) and are also able to respond to stimuli (nervous system).[34, 35] These systems have been adapting themselves from the beginning of life, and this adaptation is reflected in our daily lives today. When one is hungry, the brain expresses a need to find food. When something does not sit well in the digestive tract, the brain makes the experience quite unbearable. The connection is so deep that we even experience "gut feelings" and "butterflies in the stomach" from emotional stimuli unrelated to food.[36] We refer to this relationship as the "gut-brain axis."[37]

The Second Brain

The intestines contain the second largest network of neurons outside of the central nervous system.[38, 39] In fact, the gut is often referred to as the "second brain."[40, 41] Did you know that serotonin (a well-known neurotransmitter in the brain that is said to control everything from appetite, sleep, memory, learning and temperature regulation, to mood, behavior, cardiovascular function, muscle contraction, endocrine regulation, and depression) is found in two main locations of the human body—the brain and the gut?[42] Melatonin, a neurotransmitter associated primarily with sleep-wake cycles, is also found in these two locations.[43, 44] The gut is a concentrated area for these neurotransmitters. In fact:

About 90 percent of the body's total serotonin and at least 70 percent of its melatonin is found in the gut![45 46, 47]

This gut–brain connection is undeniable, which is empowering because there are self-actionable protocols for healing our digestion that may be the most powerful tools that we can use to optimize our health and function.

What Can Go Wrong?

A substantial list of triggers may lead to a problem with digestion known as leaky gut (or intestinal permeability), including brain injury and other neurological conditions.[48] Several studies show how important the brain-gut connection is and how neurological issues can lead to digestive problems and vice versa. Improper digestion can lead to neurological disorders as well.[49, 50, 51] This means that leaky gut contributes to brain problems and brain problems contribute to leaky gut… It's a vicious cycle that gets worse and worse if not properly addressed.

As I said, there is a long list of triggers that may lead to (or that are a symptom of) leaky gut, so let's talk about a few catalysts. Essentially, if you have ever sustained a brain injury or you have any neurological condition, then leaky gut is almost a certainty.[52, 53] Additionally, if you experience any brain-based symptoms (such as brain fog, headaches, depression, anxiety, or ADHD), then there is a strong possibility that leaky gut is a factor.[54] If you have low energy, skin problems, allergies, joint or muscle pain, experience any digestive symptoms (even as seemingly benign as passing gas or food intolerances), leaky gut is extremely likely.[55, 56]

It is also becoming clear that for any autoimmune condition to manifest into a diagnosable condition, leaky gut first needs to be present.[57, 58, 59] This means that if you have been diagnosed with Hashimoto's, rheumatoid arthritis, lupus, celiac disease, multiple sclerosis, type 1 diabetes, or any other autoimmune condition, and you have not addressed intestinal permeability (leaky gut), it is very important that you do. Let's explore this condition.

WHAT IS "LEAKY GUT?"

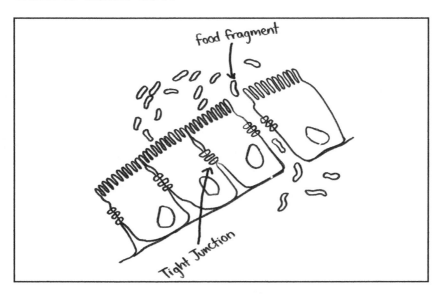

Leaky Gut Syndrome, or intestinal permeability, is a condition in which un-digested food particles cross into the bloodstream undigested, resulting in inflammation and impaired nutrient absorption.[60, 61, 62]

After I had progressed through my recovery in a dense brain fog for about ten months post-injury, the results of a blood test led me to an incredibly important realization.

This blood test examined the levels of macronutrients and other compounds in my blood, and the results demonstrated that some of my protein levels were low. This was surprising because I had meat with every meal and I had a protein shake every morning.

My body was not absorbing the protein I was eating.

It was clear that my digestion was not delivering at least some of the nutrients that my brain and body needed to repair optimally, and the work I was doing to heal myself through exercise and therapy was not being properly supported. The brain is unable to heal effectively without adequate brain-building nutrients.

Normally, food is partially digested in the stomach before moving on to the small intestine. Nutrients are then absorbed into the blood through the gut lining and transported throughout the brain and body so that they can fuel, maintain, and repair our cells.[63]

With Leaky Gut, whole food particles pass through the intestinal wall and into the blood *before* being completely broken down or digested.[64, 65] As a result, the blood does not recognize these undigested food particles and an immune response occurs just as it would if there were a splinter or any other foreign object in the bloodstream.[66, 67] This immune response causes inflammation, sending signaling molecules called cytokines to the area.[68, 69, 70]

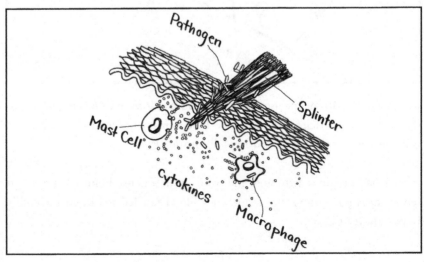

A Link to the Brain

The same glue that seals our gut is also used to seal our blood-brain-barrier, which is what keeps toxins and other cellular debris out of our brain.[71, 72] As our gut becomes leaky to undigested food particles, so does our brain to waste and other compounds that don't belong there.[73, 74] Additionally, a 1995 study from the *Journal of Neuroimmunomodulation* titled "Passage of Cytokines across the Blood-Brain Barrier" found that these inflammatory cytokines are very small and can cross even a healthy blood-brain barrier, causing inflammation in the brain.[75] The study concluded that: "evidence shows that passage of cytokines across the BBB [blood-brain barrier] occurs, providing a route by which blood-borne cytokines could potentially affect brain function."[76] This suggests that:

Even in healthy individuals, inflammation anywhere in the body could trigger inflammation in the brain. [77]

A 2003 study published in the *Proceedings of the National Academy of Sciences* is titled "Inflammation is detrimental for neurogenesis in adult brain."[78] The title says it all. Remember that neurons are the functional cells of the brain, so neurogenesis is the creation of new neurons. This article shows us that inflammation hinders the creation of new neurons.

When the brain becomes inflamed, there is a reduction in brain activity including the output of information from the brain to the digestive system.[79, 80, 81, 82] This decrease in communication may cause increased intestinal permeability (leaky gut) leading to additional inflammation and cytokines in the bloodstream, which are then able to cross the blood-brain barrier and induce even more inflammation in the brain.[83, 84, 85, 86] In other words, an inflammatory loop develops which exacerbates itself.

There are no pain receptors in the brain, and because the brain is our organ of perception, if the brain itself is inflamed, we may not notice the symptoms.[87, 88] Again, how can one tell that it's raining when underwater?

In other words, we may be experiencing inflammation in the brain without being able to perceive any brain-based symptoms or any noticeable indigestion.[89, 90]

The Inflammatory Loop of Leaky Gut

Why is the patient not digesting some nutrients?

Because the intestinal wall is permeable

Because there are many cytokines in the bloodstream

Because the brain is not communicating effectively with the gut

Because the brain is inflamed

Breaking the Loop

Did you know that the intro phase to any functional medicine protocol is to address Leaky Gut? This is because the digestive system is where we take in most substances, other than air, from the outside.

> **Everything you eat or drink is either inflammatory or anti-inflammatory.**[91]

There is almost no food or drink that is neutral except for pure water. Because the digestive system is our body's primary access point of solid and liquid matter into the body, it is also a primary site of inflammation.[92]

> **The way to break the inflammatory loop is to focus on the intestinal wall permeability (leaky gut).**[93]

This book will outline the foods and targeted nutrients that I understand to be most beneficial for the function of brain cells, which have been key to my own recovery. But remember that the brain is only able to receive the nutrition that it is able to absorb, and leaky gut can prevent us from absorbing many of the nutrients that we are ingesting. For this reason, I have also included some general guidelines for gut healing.

Keep in mind that we are all unique and additional support may be warranted. You can learn more about leaky gut and find support and other tools that are useful to optimize digestion at: feedabrain.com/digestion.

After addressing the cause, we want to quell the inflammation that has already been triggered. A lot of focus is put into developing drugs to fight inflammation, but the most important compound that acts as our natural defense against inflammation is also the same compound that is referred to as the brain and body's energy currency. This compound is known as ATP, or adenosine triphosphate.

BRAIN ENERGY & MITOCHONDRIAL FUNCTION

What is ATP?

ATP is a compound where energy is stored.[94] It is produced in the mitochondria of most cells.[95] Thinking again of each cell as a vehicle, the mitochondria would be the engine, which produces energy, or ATP, for different cellular functions. In the same way that the engine of a vehicle does more than just turn the wheels (AC, stereo, power windows, power steering, recharge your battery, etc.), ATP does more than just give you energy. ATP plays a role in most biochemical reactions in the brain and body, including reactions that quell inflammation.[96, 97, 98] We want to optimize the mitochondrial production of ATP by giving them the ingredients they need. So which nutrients play a role in mitochondrial function? A more fitting question is -- are there any nutrients that don't play a role?

The definition of a nutrient is a substance that provides nourishment that is essential for growth and the maintenance of life.[99] To grow or maintain life we need energy, and mitochondrial function is what creates that energy.[100]

When it comes to the nutrients found in food, Bruce Ames, a professor of Biochemistry and Molecular Biology Emeritus at the University of California, Berkeley, uses the term "micronutrient" to describe all the minerals, vitamins, essential fatty acids, and amino acids that play a role in biology.[101] Ames states that about 40 micronutriets are required in the human diet, but there also seem to be at least 25,000 types of phytonutrients (certain micronutrients found in plants) many of which have been shown to have some biological value.[102, 103] Again, food, in its whole food form, likely contains many other nutrients that we have not yet discovered or do not yet know the importance of, and it may be the ways in which these unrecognized nutrients work together that make such a profound impact on neurological recovery. This is going to be an underlying theme of this book and why what I have written is more a meal plan guide rather than a supplementation protocol. We want to get almost all of our nutrients in the same form as what we have evolved with, which is why we want to get these nutrients in the food we eat.

With this in mind, the next question becomes clear:

What is the optimal diet to power the cells of the brain? Soon after healing my gut, I became aware of Dr. Terry Wahls MD. Her research contributed greatly to my understanding of what I would want to eat to supply my neurons with the nutrients they craved.

Who is Dr. Terry Wahls?

In 2000, Dr. Terry Wahls was diagnosed with Multiple Sclerosis (MS), a neurodegenerative disease in which the communication of the nervous system is disrupted and progressively deteriorates.[104] This is an autoimmune disease in which the body attacks the myelin, or the fatty sheath that increases the speed of neuronal signals (which we talked about earlier).[105]

Dr. Wahls sought out the best clinics that conventional medicine had to offer, participating in many different treatments for multiple sclerosis. As Terry went to highly regarded locations to treat her condition, her children continued to see their once active, athletic mother increasingly less able to perform basic activities. Within four years, her disease progressed to the point where she needed a tilt-recline wheelchair, and she spent most her time in a zero-gravity chair.[106]

Terry knew that the way she handled this disabling condition would act as a model for her children. She wanted to set an example of perseverance and determination to overcome life's obstacles. Every night, she would search the Internet for information that might help her heal, eventually stumbling upon the Institute for Functional Medicine.[107]

The goal of the Institute for Functional Medicine is to provide a different way to care for people with chronic conditions by looking at how different biomarkers, lifestyle, and environmental factors contribute to health or disease.[108] In other words, conventional medicine seems to consider health to be the absence of injury or disease, where functional medicine aims to promote health and optimal function by supplying nutrients to the cells within the brain and body, and by removing substances that hinder health and function. Both of these paradigms have an enormous amount of value. Conventional medicine saves millions of lives (including my own) with heroic critical care, surgical intervention, and pharmaceutical relief. In addition to conventional medicine's expertise in acute care, the principles of functional medicine have been used to enhance quality of life for millions with chronic conditions such as autoimmunity, cancer, IBS, and brain injury or disease.[109]

After taking a course on neuroprotection *(Neuroprotection: A Functional Medicine Approach for Common and Uncommon Neurologic Syndromes)*, Terry began to see medicine in a new light.[110]

> **As a traditionally trained MD, she realized that her nutritional training was inadequate at best.[111]**

Even though the average American Medical Doctor (MD) spends about 14 years training for the job (four years of college, four years of medical school, and residencies and fellowships that last between three and eight years), a medical doctor in the US only receives about 24 hours of nutrition training.[112] This means that it is likely that less than 0.01 percent of an MD's classroom training is spent on nutrition. Additionally, the nutrition training from American medical schools has been in line with the nutritional guidelines of the United States Department of Agriculture (USDA) for decades, and there are many strong arguments pointing out how these guidelines have been contributing to the decline of America's health.[113]

Terry's newfound outlook on nutrition set her on a path which included a long list of food-based supplements and a daily regimen. Although it wasn't the way she had been trained, Terry began to treat her own condition by using supplements to support the metabolism of her cells with specific enzymes, amino acids, vitamins, minerals, antioxidants, fatty acids, and other compounds that had been shown in peer-reviewed studies to support the cellular metabolism of the nervous system.[114]

As the weeks passed, her condition began to slightly improve. But as an open-minded MD, Terry was aware that, while our scientific advances are continually expanding, there is a great deal we do not yet know. She reasoned that there must be many nutrients that we do not yet know the importance of, or that we have not yet discovered.[115] And because nutrients are not found in nature in isolated pill form, Terry had the insight to take this list of nutritional supplements and to learn where they were in the foods that were available to her.[116]

Cells need the right fuel to function properly, and this cellular fuel comes from food.[117]

She needed an eating plan that would maximize her brain cell function. By incorporating functional medicine concepts, principles of evolutionary biology, and ideas that were born out of her own research, Terry set out to create an eating plan to regain her nervous system function.[118]

After countless hours spent researching and organizing thoughts, Terry now had a collection of foods to add to her diet that seemed to match up nutritionally to the list of supplements that she had been using.[119] This, she says, is "when things really began to change in [her] brain and body."[120]

After just three months on this new diet, as well as a specific regimen of different exercises, she went from a tilt-recline wheelchair to being able to *walk* from exam rooms using only one cane. After six months, she could walk around the entire hospital without a cane.[121]

She now enjoys hiking with her family and recently completed an 18-mile bike ride![122]

In her book, *The Wahls Protocol*, she explains how she beats MS with diet, lifestyle, and targeted therapies, and she lays out a nutritional protocol for others to follow for their own health.[123] You can learn more about Dr. Wahls at feedabrain.com/terry.

How Does That Apply to My Brain?

You may wonder what Dr. Terry Wahls' story of healing from the effects of Multiple Sclerosis has to do with our brain function or repair. As I mentioned before, what it all comes down to is the health of the living cell. Because the cells within the central nervous system are what have been affected in both of our ailments, it does not matter that Terry, myself, or those with other neurological disorders have very different conditions. Whether the condition is a neurodegenerative disease or brain injury, the nutritional support for brain cells (neurons and glia), is universally needed. As discussed earlier, inflammation anywhere in the body may inflame the brain, so by implementing nutritional changes to support brain health, we will also be supporting overall health.[124]

After my injury, I needed to find a way to support the health of my neurons and glia nutritionally, and Terry's research and publications acted as an amazing roadmap towards my recovery. She had the brilliance, the motivation, and the resources to figure out how to supply the cells of her brain with the best and most effective nutrition to function, and she had written a book about her experience, *The Wahls Protocol*.[125]

Among other important therapies, I included many aspects of Dr. Wahls' nutritional protocol in the recovery of my brain and body. I saw the positive difference these nutritional changes made in me. In an effort to help others attain results and improve their lives, I have included in this book many of the nutritional tools that I have learned to optimize brain function and repair. I am delighted and honored to say that Dr. Wahls has been very supportive in my journey to bring this book into existence in order to get this information into the hands of you, your family, or your patients.

Chapter 3
THE INS AND OUTS OVERVIEW

WHAT TO INCLUDE & EXCLUDE FROM OUR DIETS

Many popular diets focus on restriction, caloric limitation, or avoidance of certain food types. Commonly, their strategy hinges on the demonization of nutrients like fats or carbohydrates, or entire food groups, like meat, dairy, or grains.[126]

While it is important to steer clear of foods that will undermine our success ("The Outs"), this book is more focused on including the foods we want in our diet ("The Ins"). After including the foods we want in our diet, little room will be left for the small list of foods to avoid or eliminate, anyway.

Let's begin with a bird's-eye view of the Feed a Brain meal plan. Once we address some common dietary limitations, we'll dive into the specifics of how and why the dietary changes outlined in these pages supply the brain with the nutrients we want for optimal brain function and repair.

VEGANS AND VEGETARIANS

Most vegetarians and vegans tend to be very conscious about the effects of their food choices on the environment, on their bodies, and on the ethical treatment of animals. This is a consciousness that I share and respect, as I have become more aware of how food affects our physiology. I also wrestle with the unsustainable and unethical treatment of factory farmed animals.[127] Unfortunately, a strict vegan or vegetarian diet, unless carefully practiced and supplemented, often results in deficiencies of some important nutrients like vitamin B12, calcium, iron, zinc, EPA, DHA, and other nutrients that many experts agree are needed for brain recovery, repair, and optimization.[128, 129, 130, 131]

While I completely understand and respect the choice to not eat animals for ethical reasons, if the choice is influenced heavily by optimal nutrition, please read on with an open mind and heart as we explore the types of foods that research has shown to best support the nervous system.

The most important nutrient that is rarely supplied adequately in a vegetarian or vegan diet is DHA (a kind of Omega-3 fatty acid that is largely found in cold water fish like mackerel, sardines, salmon, and tuna).

DHA Use in Treating TBI

Even though the use of DHA has not yet become a standard part of clinical practice, research showing the importance of this nutrient to brain health and repair is becoming more widely understood.

As you will see, **DHA has been shown to be extremely useful towards TBI recovery and neuroprotection (the resilience and preservation of neuronal structure and/or function).**

After finding very favorable results in a study testing the use of DHA *after* a severe traumatic brain injury (diffuse axonal injury) in rats,[132] the West Virginia University School of Medicine conducted a follow-up study to see the effect of DHA supplementation *before* a brain injury. The study found that rats who were supplemented with DHA before a brain injury showed less damage done to the brain after, as well as better brain function, as assessed by maze testing.[133]

Omega-3s have also been used in humans to treat traumatic brain injury. One such study in the *American Journal of Emergency Medicine* presents a case study about a teenager who sustained a severe TBI in 2010.[134] Like me, he was diagnosed with a diffuse axonal injury with an initial Glasgow Coma Score of 3, which is the lowest possible score (no response to any stimuli, but still alive). Thought to be in a permanent vegetative state, he was given a gastric tube (PEG), and a procedure was performed which left him breathing through a tube protruding from his neck (tracheotomy).[135]

Ten days after the injury, he was given a large dose (15 ml, which is about 13g) twice a day of Nordic Natural Ultimate Omega via his PEG (feeding tube). On the 21st day, he was weaned off the ventilator, and soon progressed from a vegetative state to attending his high school graduation three months later![136]

Information on the product used in this case study, and other high quality fish oils like it, can be found at feedabrain.com/omega.

Is There a Vegetarian Source of DHA?

DHA is considered a "conditionally essential" Omega-3 fatty acid, meaning that our bodies can create this important fatty acid from other nutrients, but the conversion of almost all vegetarian sources of Omega-3s to DHA is not efficient. For example, flax, walnut, mustard seed oil, and other vegetarian sources of omega 3s do not actually contain any DHA, only the precursor to DHA (ALA).[137] In biochemistry, a precursor refers to a substance that can be used to make another. This means that ALA can be used to make DHA, but, unfortunately, even the ability of healthy people to convert ALA to DHA is estimated to be only 0.2% to 4%.[138]

Our body's poor means of converting most vegetarian sources of Omega-3 fatty acids to DHA seem only to be in place as a backup to getting this nutrient directly from animal sources.[139] Luckily for strict vegans and vegetarians, there does seem to be a possible vegan supplement of actual DHA. This source is derived from algae and may provide the same benefits of animal sourced DHA, though further research is needed.[140, 141, 142] You can find more information on this vegan source of DHA at feedabrain.com/vegan.

As you can see, DHA is incredibly important and, without targeted supplementation, DHA is scarce in a vegan or vegetarian diet. I encourage fish consumption and/or supplementation of fish oils for this nutrient.

Some vegans and vegetarians choose to supply this nutrient by supplementing with algae oil. Others have made the decision to take the higher-dose and less expensive DHA content available by supplementing with a high DHA fish oil. Still others have made the difficult decision to change their ideology and move away from vegan or vegetarianism by switching to a pescatarian diet (diet including fish) with fatty fish like tuna and salmon. Information on algae based vegan DHA supplements can be found at feedabrain.com/vegan.

Information on high-quality mail order frozen or canned fish can be found at feedabrain.com/fish. Information on recommended fish oils can be found at feedabrain.com/omega.

While I regularly eat vegan fare, I am not and never have been a vegan or vegetarian. Therefore, my experience with these dietary practices, while still supplying brain building nutrition, is limited. While I will be providing some supplementation alternatives, a vegan or vegetarian meal plan is beyond the scope of this book. If a vegan or vegetarian diet is desired, it is advised that you take this book to your dietitian to develop a meal plan that still supplies enough of these foods to make a strong impact on neurological health.

OUTLINING THESE NUTRITIONAL GUIDELINES
The primary nutritional objective of this book is to provide practices that can be used to incorporate certain kinds of fruits, vegetables, and meats, as well as fats and other nutrient-dense ingredients that improve brain health and function. Whether eating conventionally or through a gastric tube, this book will supply recipe guidelines that will help the brain get the nutrition it needs to best support the nervous system.

Our meals and smoothies will consist of vegetables, fruits, healthy fats, and protein (mostly from animals and fish). We will incorporate soups, stews, salads and smoothies which can be eaten whole, pureed, or fed via a gastric tube. This gives families with members who are not eating conventionally an opportunity to eat the same meals together, which helps to bring some normalcy to family dinners.

Let's start with a simple outline of the foods we want to add, avoid, and completely remove so that we can begin to wrap our head around the concepts as they are later explained. First, we will look at the foods that we want to avoid, and then we will address the two foods that we will need to temporarily remove completely, why we want to remove them, and how we can keep them out of our diets. Foods that are removed from this meal plan should be removed 100% for at least 60 days. Foods that are to be avoided can be consumed in small quantities, but they should be avoided because they are not nutrition for optimal brain function and repair. Though they are "allowed," we want to leave as much room as we can for foods that will supply our brains with the best nutrition. After covering the foods we will be removing or avoiding, the bulk of this book will cover what foods supply nutrition for optimal brain function and repair, why we want enough of them, and how we can pack all of these supportive nutrients into our diets.

Often, when we are given instructions without understanding why, it feels as if we are following the instructions for no reason other than that we have been asked. When we have a better understanding of why we are making certain changes, we are empowered to take our health and recovery into our own hands.

An Outline to the Feed a Brain Meal Plan

There will be several reference charts throughout this book, and I recommend that you print them out and put them on your fridge or somewhere else that is easy to reference while preparing food. Questions tend to come up when our hands are full, we're short on time, and/or we're just too hungry to find this information and to sift through it for the simple answer. Being able to simply glance at an image or chart to get an answer prevents us from making assumptions or giving up.

Even though what we will be limiting or removing from our diet is not the focus of this book, in order for us to reap the benefits of the brain building nutrients that we will be providing ("The Ins"), we first need to remove the foods that will stand in the way of our progress ("The Outs").

If we continue to eat foods that are inflammatory to us, even if we bring in all the right nutrients and anti-inflammatory compounds, the damage that these inflammatory foods are doing will only be slowed. Think of it like this: If every morning we slam our thumb in our desk drawer, it doesn't matter how many painkillers, anti-inflammatories, topical ointments, fancy Band-Aids, or nutritional support protocols we provide; our thumb will not heal until we stop slamming it in the drawer. Let's stop slamming our thumbs in drawers! Let's remove or reduce inflammatory foods from our diets.

The first handout that I would like you to print out or view online is an over-view of the foods we want to include and exclude from our diets in order to heal and to optimize our brains ("The Ins & Outs: What to Include and Exclude").

The handouts are generally too detailed to reproduce very clearly in this book, so go to feedabrain.com/handouts to pull up the handouts on your computer or smartphone in a full -size color PDF document.

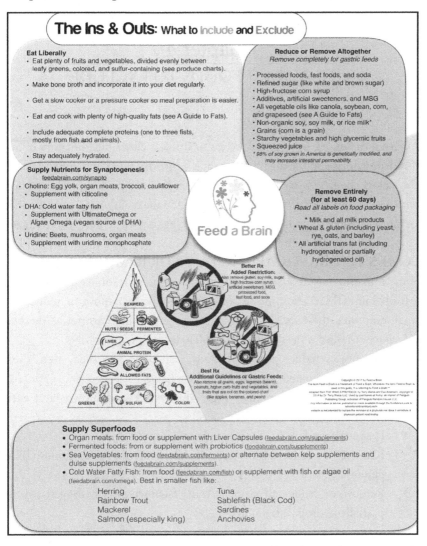

Adapted from THE WAHLS PROTOCOL by Terry Wahls and Eve Adamson, copyright ©2014 by Dr. Terry Wahls L.LC. Used by permission of Avery, an imprint of Penguin Publishing Group, a division of Penguin Random House LLC.

*For your convenience, all charts can be found as printable, full-size, color PDF files at feedabrain.com/handouts.

Chapter 4
THE OUTS — FOODS TO EXCLUDE

As stated earlier, everything that we eat or drink is either inflammatory or anti-inflammatory, and the digestive system is a primary site of inflammation. We also talked about how studies show that, even in healthy adults, inflammation *anywhere* in the body can trigger inflammation in the brain. And, especially after an injury, inflammation in the brain is something that we do *not* want to trigger.

FOODS TO DRASTICALLY REDUCE OR REMOVE

Some inflammatory foods need little explanation. Still, some other foods are less obvious. These are some inflammatory foods to remove or reduce. In small amounts, these do not seem to be as potentially harmful as the two substances that we want to eliminate 100% (at least temporarily):

- Remove or reduce processed foods, fast foods, and soda, even "diet" soda (unsweetened sparkling water is okay).
- Remove or reduce refined sugar (like white and brown, and even "natural" sugar).
- Remove or reduce high-fructose corn syrup.[143]
- Remove or reduce additives, artificial sweeteners, and monosodium glutamate.[144, 145]
- Remove or reduce all artificial trans fat, including hydrogenated, or partially hydrogenated oil.[146]

Some less well known inflammatory foods should also be reduced or removed.

- Remove or reduce all vegetable oils like canola, soybean, corn, and grapeseed oils.[147, 148, 149]
- Remove or reduce non-organic soy or soy milk (98% of soy grown in America is genetically modified, and may increase intestinal permeability).[150]

FOODS TO COMPLETELY REMOVE
(For at Least 60 Days)

We have only two foods that must be strictly eliminated from our diets, at least temporarily:

- Remove wheat and any product that includes wheat, wheat flour, yeast, rye, oats, or barley (unless labeled "gluten free").
- Remove milk (and milk products like cream, yogurt, butter, cheese, ice cream, frozen yogurt etc.).

In my work with one of the best functional nutritionists and health educators, Andrea Nakayama, I have learned of so many different therapeutic and nutritional guidelines and recommendations. It has become very apparent that we are all different or bio-individual. Foods that are well tolerated by me may not be well tolerated by you. However, two of the foods that are removed, at least temporarily, from *every* single anti-inflammatory protocol that I have seen are wheat and milk (specifically gluten and casein, proteins found in wheat and milk).

I completely understand that these suggestions may be upsetting to hear, but I would like you to do yourself a favor and to stop eating wheat and milk today. Do it cold turkey, and do it 100%. This may be the most important thing we can do for our health. We can try reintroducing these foods, one at a time, after 60 days to see how they are tolerated in our bodies, but we can thrive without them. An amazingly effective method that can be used to curb cravings for foods that are not part of this meal plan is by consuming exogenous ketones, which we will talk about later.

Why Wheat and Milk?

When writing what would become the first draft of this book, I was helping guide a brain injury survivor and her family to eat better for brain health. As I wrote, I recalled the difficulties I had giving up some foods, even if it was temporary. My functional neurologist told me that these foods could get in the way of my recovery, and I wanted to give my brain the best shot, so I did what he said... I removed the foods I was told to, limited others, and I soon began to replace those foods with plenty of what I found to be the right nutrition for my brain (outlined in "The Ins" chapters).

There are many delicious alternatives to milk and milk products. Some examples include almond milk, coconut milk, cashew milk, macadamia milk, etc. There are great yogurts made from the same types of milk listed.

There are also many "gluten free" alternatives to wheat products, but keep in mind that most of these alternatives are made from other grains or from nuts, and we want to limit all nuts and grains to leave room for the brain building nutrients outlined in "The Ins" chapters.

I remember being angry about giving up these two foods which I loved. I mean, I am a third-generation Italian who grew up with his grandma's pasta, loads of parmesan, and lasagna. In fact, when I could eat again after not being able to swallow for months, my grandma's pasta was one of the first foods that I requested. It was only later that I saw the power of food for brain health. The reason we want to remove these two foods is because they are widely considered to be the two most inflammatory foods that most of us regularly consume.

Because of the fogging effect of inflammatory foods and leaky gut, we may be experiencing inflammation in the brain from wheat and milk without being able to perceive any brain-based symptoms or any noticeable indigestion.[151, 152] The effects of wheat and milk go far beyond digestive problems.[153] Let's take a look at the research for each.

Wheat (gluten): There are countless studies concerning immune responses to wheat and gluten,[154, 155] but this one especially caught my attention. In early 2015, a study conducted by the University of Maryland showed that ingested gliadin (the water soluble portion of wheat) leads to increased leaky gut in *all humans*.[156] The exact words in the conclusion said: "increased intestinal permeability after gliadin exposure occurs in all individuals."[157]

Removing, or at least drastically limiting, the wheat in your diet may be the most important thing you can do to nutritionally support your brain health and recovery!

There are several excellent guides and courses to help you transition to a gluten free lifestyle (see feedabrain.com/gluten), but the basic principle is to remove wheat, yeast, rye, oats (unless marked gluten free), and barley (think "WhY ROB"… Like "Why rob your body of nutrients?"). The hardest part in removing gluten is being a detective when it comes to hidden sources like sauces, soups, condiments, and so much more (which we are about to discuss). For 60 days, try to eat only whole foods like meat, fruits, and vegetables.

Milk (casein and lactose): Lactose intolerance is not the only kind of intolerance that we can have to milk. In addition to the sugar found in milk (lactose), an immune response is commonly also triggered by six different milk proteins (four casein and two whey).[158, 159] While there is less research on casein, lactose, and whey, milk is widely considered to be the second most inflammatory food in our modern diet (second only to gluten).[160,]

Speaking from my own experience, as a child, I was lactose intolerant before I grew out of it and, as an adult, I no longer had a noticeable reaction. In fact, just the day before my injury, I had a slice of New York pizza from my local pizza shop (wheat and milk), which I went to just about every day without a noticeable reaction. After my brain injury, I noticed more mucus production and I felt groggy when I had milk or cheese, even without the wheat. It turns out that certain proteins found in wheat and milk (gliadin and casein) are molecularly similar which is likely why their effects in the brain and body are also similar.[161, 162]

Giving up the "Comfort Foods"

Wheat and milk products are considered "comfort foods" for a reason (think mac and cheese, pizza, quesadilla or chicken fried steak with cream gravy). It appears that both wheat (gluten) and dairy (casein) proteins have an opiate-like, addictive effect in the brain.[163] This is why giving them up can actually feel like withdrawal. I completely realize that if you and/or your loved one is currently eating these foods, giving them up is easier said than done.

As we discussed, people with brain injuries/concussions[164] or brain disease,[165] as well as those who have been hospitalized and put on multiple medications and antibiotics[166, 167] are more likely to have a leaky gut. And with a leaky gut, wheat and milk can be especially damaging.[168] When wheat (gluten) and/or milk (casein) proteins get into the bloodstream undigested, the intestine becomes even more permeable, allowing other foods that weren't bothersome before to cross into the bloodstream and to also cause an immune response. This phenomenon is called cross-reactivity, which can cause an immune response to tree nuts, citrus, strawberries, or so many other foods.[169, 170, 171] This happens because the intestinal wall becomes permeable to other food particles as well, and the blood is not able to recognize any undigested food.[172]

Hang in there, because once you get past the initial phase of removing these addictive substances, your brain will be able to further heal.

Allergy Testing

Allergy testing may not show an allergy to gluten, lactose, casein, or whey; however, allergy testing does not address all of the possible responses that someone may have to a specific food.[173] Some allergy testing looks at one half of the immune system while other testing observes the other half of the immune system, but Dr. Terry Wahls points out that no test addresses both at the same time, which is what is necessary to effectively rule out an allergy or immune reaction.[174] This means that you may test negative for the few possible reactions that the test screens for when you very well could be having an immune response that is of a type that the test does not screen for. Because of this, allergy testing often results in a "false negative," meaning that the test results indicate there is no reaction when in fact there is one.[175] Therefore, Dr. Wahls says that no allergy testing offers a reliable way of knowing what foods create problems, and it is more useful to follow an elimination diet.[176]

The gold standard three-step elimination diet is used by many functional practitioners. Here's how it's done:

1. The food needs to be removed 100% for at least 60 days, but it may take up to 90 days for any possible immune response to subside.
2. The next step is to reintroduce the food in a substantial amount for a few days and to observe any possible changes in feeling, mucus or saliva secretion, trouble breathing, brain function, anxiety, temper, pain, digestive symptoms, or any other change that occurs, even if seemingly unrelated (an immune response can show itself in any number of possible ways).
3. If you notice an effect through this experiment, the food likely creates an inflammatory response at that time. You may want to wait 30 days more than the last removal period and then to try again (immune

reactions can sometimes subside) or simply remove the food from your diet. I still recommend removing, or drastically limiting, both wheat and milk long term because of the above studies.

We also need to pay attention to the ingredients of sauces, toothpastes, deodorants, soaps, skincare products, etc. Wheat and milk containing products are found in many places that most of us would never think. Double check these kinds of products for common inflammatory compounds like gluten, dairy, and egg (all products found on feedabrain.com are free of gluten and potentially harmful proteins found in dairy and egg):

- Sunscreens and lotions.
- Shampoos, conditioners, cosmetics, and styling products.
- Lip balm and glosses.
- Spices, salad dressing, dip, and soup mixes.
- Imitation crab (may include eggs and/or gluten).
- Beer (most beer is made with wheat, yeast, rye, oats, and/or barley).
- Worcestershire, soy, BBQ, and other sauces.
- Play Dough (sometimes made with wheat flour).
- Vitamins, supplements, and medications.[177]

Keep in mind that we will be able to reintroduce these foods after 60 days and will then be able to choose whether it is worth it to have a little. I, for example, love cheese, and I have not yet found a cheese alternative that does it for me. Additionally, while I don't eat bread or have anything made with dough that is not gluten-free, I no longer need to worry too much about trace amounts of gluten, yeast, rye, oats, or barley in my food. So even though I experience an immune response from wheat and milk, it's not so bad that I need to remove the food entirely or to stress myself out about small exposure to these inflammatory foods because I've already done the work healing my leaky gut. At this point, I allow myself to have a bit from time to time.

I did the work at first and eliminated all wheat and dairy for well over 60 days. The several months of complete elimination of these foods may be necessary for us to notice our symptoms, and noticing our symptoms is a good thing. Again, how can one tell that it's raining when under water? Remember that the brain is our organ of perception, so when the brain itself is inflamed, we may not notice brain-based symptoms.[178, 179] However, for optimal brain function and repair, we want to be fully aware of how foods make us feel, and these foods are considered by many researchers to be the biggest triggers of brain inflammation.[180, 181] Dr. Kharrazian is so sure about the effect of gluten on the brain that he wrote in his brain book, *Why Isn't My Brain Working?*, that "[i]f you have a confirmed gluten sensitivity and feel going gluten free is too difficult, it is time for you to put this book down and realize your brain has no chance and you will continue to get worse."[182]

While we need to break our dependence on certain foods in the short term, our long-term relationship with food should not be one of deprivation, even if we need to completely remove a certain food forever. We can reframe our relationship to foods that do not help our brains as something that does not give to us, but that takes from us. Let's find a place where we can optimize our brain function and repair while still enjoying our food. Remember, the healthiest thing we can do for our brain is to enjoy our life and to do so sustainably. Long-term deprivation is not the goal.

Today my dietary "restrictions" are not strict limitations on what I can eat. My dietary "restrictions" are *my choice* for better brain health. I now have the wiggle room to occasionally eat foods that are known to be inflammatory for me, and do so with the knowledge of my own intolerance to them. I am now able to recognize how foods affect me. I choose to eat mostly foods that support my brain and to drastically limit those that seem to be harmful to it.

While I was in the early stages of nutritionally supporting my recovering brain, no matter how much I wanted to "cheat," I had to understand that I would only be cheating myself. It felt like deprivation for a few weeks, but eventually I could not deny that my brain was showing signs of improved function. My thinking was clearer, I was communicating more effectively, and my mood had improved. It no longer felt like deprivation. It was now my choice for better brain health. Not only did this meal plan eventually become easier, but I learned more recipes and ideas to supply these nutrients, and it actually became fun. I was getting more of my brain and abilities back each day! I was healing myself through nutrition, which was empowering!

I held the keys to my own brain health...
and you hold the keys to yours.

Chapter 5
THE INS — BONE BROTH

Now that we have addressed the small list of foods to avoid, and the two foods that we want to eliminate, it's time we talk about the important foods that will support our brain health. Let's start with an especially powerful ingredient for healing our guts and supporting our skin and tissue health. This ingredient can act as a base for many of our meals.

SOUP FOR THE SOUL: CREATING KILLER BROTH

"Good broth will resurrect the dead."
- South American proverb

Bones and Minerals

For months after my injury, I woke up every morning in immense pain. It was a pain unlike any I had ever experienced. My legs tingled like they were numb, yet they throbbed. My bones ached like I was a century old. In fact, I morbidly joked by calling my brain injury "instant old man." When I didn't exercise during the day or stretch before bed, the pain that I would wake up to the next morning was excruciating, and it was not getting any better.

As my brain fog continued to dissipate, I began studying functional nutrition and learned how beneficial bone broth, or homemade stock, could be for the health of our cells. This was not the kind of broth I had been using from a can or box my whole life, but the kind of broth my grandma made from scratch.

Why Don't I Just Buy Broth from a Can or Box?

I admit that I was a bit skeptical that homemade stock (bone broth) would be so beneficial, and homemade broth seemed intimidating, but it turned out that making traditional broth is actually very simple, much tastier, and less expensive than store bought broth. I was soon implementing homemade bone broth into my diet every day.

With the initial sip from my first batch, I felt as if every cell in my body was thanking me. I ended up making soup and having a few more mugs of broth that day, and the next morning, for the first time in months, I woke up without feeling like an old man. My pain had reduced, and the tingling had almost vanished. Amazed, I began to research why this practice could possibly have such a powerful effect.

Stock made the traditional way has been shown to be beneficial for many reasons, and one of these reasons is its mineral content. Minerals are like spark plugs for our metabolism and physiology. They are the catalysts to many biological functions, especially nervous system functions, neurotransmitter production, and muscle contraction.[183, 184, 185] In addition to important minerals, homemade stock also contains collagen, gelatin, glycine, proline, and other nutrients that are important for joint, vision, heart, and brain health.[186, 187, 188]

There are some great articles about cooking with bones which you can find at feedabrain.com/bones, but if you don't want to, or don't have the time to make your own broth, you can find information on sources of pre-made high quality bone broth at feedabrain.com/broth.

Where Do I Get Bones and What Do I Do With Them?

Bones may be purchased for very little cost by asking the butcher at just about any grocery store. We can use the bones from any edible animal, and any bone will do. Butchers almost always have beef bones. Grass-fed beef or buffalo bones or pasture-raised pigs, chicken, or turkey bones make an even healthier broth, but don't let the absence of a grass-fed, organic, or pasture raised label keep you from making this protocol a part of your healing practice.[189] If you roast a whole chicken, save the bones. Bones from a store-bought rotisserie chicken can also be used. If you have a dish at a restaurant that has bones, ask to take them home. The amount of bones needed is probably less than you think. When I first started making broth, I kept it mild. I separated the bones into sandwich baggies, each with only about a handful of bones, and I threw the bags I was not using immediately in the freezer. Each handful of bones made about six quarts of broth, but I soon developed a craving for a richer broth.

We can make broth on the stovetop, but this process is easier if we use a slow cooker or pressure cooker. You can find good examples of these appliances at feedabrain.com/tools. Let's start with a simple bare bones (no pun intended) method that I still use for chicken stock to deliver all of these nutrients. I'll then tell you the more delicious, and slightly more labor-intensive method that I use for a tastier beef broth. Here's what to do:

1. Throw some bones (a lot for a richer broth, or as little as a handful) in the pot of your cooker and fill with water.
2. Add salt, pepper, and or vinegar or a tablespoon of lemon juice (for better nutrient extraction).
3. Switch the slow cooker on low for at least six, but usually 12 or more hours, or set the pressure cooker to two to four hours on high.
4. Feel free to add fresh herbs and/or veggies to the pot for less than a quarter of the total cook time. Some examples include bay leaves, shallots, onions, carrots, celery stalks, rosemary, or thyme.
5. Use tongs to remove the solids from the cooker and then strain broth.
6. Cool the broth quickly by adding ice or return the strained broth to the slow cooker or pressure cooker.
7. If cooling broth, distribute broth into smaller containers and store in fridge or freezer (frozen broth will expand, so leave room for this to avoid breaking or shattering storage container). If returning strained broth to cooker, set to the warm setting and let the broth sit available for a week or so.

There are recipes all over the internet, but this is the chicken broth recipe that I regularly use.

*This and other recipes can be found at feedabrain.com/recipes.

BONE BROTH INSPIRED BY V
(PALEOBOSSLADY.COM)

Yield: 6 servings
Prep Time: 5 minutes
Cook Time: 2.5-24 hours (depending on equipment)

Ingredients:

1 lbs chicken feet (or another kind of bones)
1 lbs chicken back/neck (or other kind of bones)
1 tablespoon organic apple cider vinegar
6-10 quarts water (preferably filtered or spring)
optional - 2 bay leaves
optional - 1 teaspoon of whole cloves
optional - 1 unpeeled shallot or ½ onion
optional - 2-5 unpeeled carrots
optional - 2-5 celery stalks with leaves
optional - 1 bunch of fresh herbs (rosemary, thyme, and/or sage)
optional - ½ - 2 tbsp salt to taste (preferably pink Himalayan sea salt)
optional - ½ - 2 tbsp black pepper to taste (preferably fresh ground)

Preparations:

1. Put the first 6 ingredients (all except the salt, pepper, fresh herbs, and vegetables) into a slow cooker or pressure cooker).
2. Set slow cooker to the low setting for 8-20 hours. (in pressure cooker, set on high for 2-4 hours)
3. Add the fresh herbs, salt and pepper to taste, and continue to cook on low for 2 more hours (in pressure cooker add vegetables, salt, pepper, and fresh herbs and set for 10 minutes)
4. Use tongs to remove large solids and then strain broth.
5. Use storage instructions below.

The more advanced method that I use on beef and other large mammal bones involves a few more steps, but the flavor is worth it, especially after getting the hang of the easier version (which I still use for chicken broth). These are the recipe guidelines I use:

1. Preheat the oven to 450 degrees F (232 degree C)
2. Blanch the bones (put the bones in boiling water) for about 20 min. Again, you may use a lot of bones for a richer broth, or as little as a handful.
3. Strain the bones and use tongs to place them separated on a cookie sheet.
4. Roast in the roaring hot 450° F oven for 20-30 min.
5. Use tongs to place the bones in your cooker (for more flavor, scrape the drippings from the bottom of the pan and add to the cooker)
6. Add water and switch the slow cooker on low for at least six, but usually 12 or more hours, or set the pressure cooker to two to four hours on high.
7. Feel free to add a few choice spices and/or veggies to the pot for less than a quarter of the total cook time (or an additional 5 min in the pressure cooker).
8. Use tongs to remove the solids from the cooker and then strain broth. You may want to hold onto the bones for the next batch. You can reuse bones to make multiple batches of broth until the bones go soft.

Storage Instructions:

You can cool the broth quickly by adding a few cups of ice. When the broth is tolerable to touch for a few seconds, store in fridge or distribute in containers to be frozen. Alternatively, you can simply set the slow cooker or pressure cooker to the warm setting and let the strained broth sit available for a week or so. In many restaurants, there is always a pot on the burner on low, providing a "master stock." This broth may be several days old, but because the pot is kept warm, the stock is enhanced as time passes.

When I find myself using less than half of my stock each time I take some, I replace the broth that I use with fresh water because Dr. Wahls has told me that she doesn't think the broth will be diluted enough to make a big difference in the nutrient content. If using most of the broth, I may still replace the broth with water, but I will then return the used bones to the pot and set the slow cooker on low overnight (or cook in pressure cooker for 5 min). My stock pot (slow cooker) is always warm to drink from or to cook with, and every week, I make a new broth with new ingredients.

Chapter 6
THE INS — PRODUCE FOR A
HEALTHY BRAIN

Now let's talk about produce. For an average-size adult male who is moderately active, the base of our meal plan is going to be three different types of produce, two to three cups of each daily. Together, these different kinds of produce give our neurons most of the ingredients for optimal brain function. I want to recognize Dr. Terry Wahls at the beginning of this chapter because her research on these categories and combinations of produce is a large part of what I share here. Her work paved the way to better brain health for us all!

FISTS OF FOLIAGE: MEASURING PORTIONS

Because there are hundreds of variables that may play a part in someone's estimated nutrient requirements, this guide does not attempt to provide the precise amounts that may be right for each person.*

If specific amounts are advised due to health concerns, they should be guided by a functional nutritionist, dietitian, doctor, or other qualified healthcare provider.

For simplicity's sake, I like to measure amounts based on the size of the individual's hand formed into a closed fist.

For the daily intake of produce, we will be consuming the equivalent of the volume of six to nine fists each day. Again, we want to evenly separate the produce into three different categories, so we are going to shoot for about two to three fists of each. But remember, this amount is a ballpark estimate dependent on many factors including macronutrient ratios, which we will talk about soon. Before we drop into the categories of these fruits and vegetables,

it is important to understand that corn is a grain and should be avoided or removed.

So what are these three categories? Let's take a look.

TWO TO THREE FISTS OF
TIGHTLY PACKED LEAFY GREENS

Let's start with the leafy greens. You know what I'm talking about—the greens in a salad that many children refuse to eat. These include arugula, collard greens, kale, spinach, herbs like cilantro, basil, or mint, as well as all types of deep-green, bright green, or red leaf lettuce (not iceberg).[190] A more comprehensive list can be found below, in the first produce chart, but I am first going to explain why we want these different types of produce.

Leafy greens are excellent sources of nutrients. In fact, vitamins B, A, C, and K are all found in leafy greens.

Vitamin B

B vitamins are important for energy, and energy is needed for the nervous system to function or to repair. In addition, folate (vitamin B9) is used to make myelin, the sheath that is wrapped around axons.[191] This sheath helps to efficiently transmit information from one part of the brain to another, or from the brain to a part of the body.[192] Without this insulation, brain function is slow.

Vitamin A

Leafy greens contain alpha- and beta-carotene, precursors to the active form of vitamin A called retinol.[193] As the name would suggest, retinol is an important nutrient for the retina.[194] And, while the retina is located at the very back of each eyeball, believe it or not, the retina is a part of the brain! Not only does retinol support the health of the retina, but it also supports bone growth, reproduction, and the health of the optic nerve in the brain.[195, 196]

Vitamin C

When it comes to immunity, vitamin C is crucial, as it has been shown to stimulate both the production and function of immune cells.[197, 198] Most animals create their own vitamin C, but humans cannot, so we must incorporate it into our diet.[199] And that's okay because it's in a lot of foods that we enjoy eating, including leafy greens.

Vitamin K

Because Vitamin K is hard to find in other foods, vitamin K may be the most important nutrient that we get from leafy greens. Vitamin K is not only very good for overall health, promoting healthy digestion and keeping blood vessels and heart valves healthy, but it is also important in the production of myelin, the nerve cell insulation that we talked about earlier. [200] Again, myelin is important for efficient communication in the nervous system.

Remember, nutrients taken in pill form are probably not as beneficial as those found in the food we eat. For example, a whole orange has over 200 phytonutrients, flavonoids, and antioxidant effects,[201] where a vitamin C supplement has only one isolated nutrient: vitamin C. Again, it may be the ways in which these other compounds work together that make such a profound impact on neurological recovery. What we do know is that whatever these nutrients are, they have many health benefits.

TWO TO THREE FISTS OF SULFUR-RICH VEGETABLES

Sulfur-rich vegetables are probably the most under-appreciated, yet hugely important foods that we will be adding to our diets. While we hear about the health benefits of some sulfur-rich foods like broccoli, Brussels sprouts, and garlic, there are so many other sulfur containing vegetables, like onions, turnips, and radishes, which don't get much press.[202]

> **Sulfur is hugely important for liver detoxification and the health of our blood vessels.**[203]

The Importance of Liver Detox

When dealing with injury or disease,[204] leaky gut, [205] or even when under stress, [206] we may be dealing with an elevated inflammatory cytokine count in the bloodstream. Not only are these cytokines small enough to cross the blood-brain barrier and inflame the brain, but like all other substances in our blood, cytokines need to be detoxified in the liver.[207] Additionally, when we use an over the counter or pharmaceutical medication, drink alcohol, or use another substance recreationally, it also needs to be filtered through the liver to be eliminated.[208] We want our detoxification pathways in the best shape possible, so we want to supply these important sulfur-rich foods.

There are 400 miles worth of blood vessels in the brain alone, and sulfur-rich vegetables also support the health of our blood vessels.[209, 210] Blood transports nutrients to different parts of the brain, and healthy blood vessels mean efficient circulation.[211] If blood circulation isn't happening at an optimal level, the brain is being deprived of important nutrients. Additionally, its ability to take away waste products is impaired, causing the brain to slowly deteriorate.[212]

Imagine if your house or apartment no longer had running water and your sink, shower, and toilet wouldn't drain. By eating sulfur-rich veggies, we are basically cleaning the plumbing that keeps our brains and bodies working, and we want to make sure our plumbing is efficiently moving nutrients in and waste out.

Sulfur-rich vegetables also keep us looking young by supporting healthy skin, hair, and nails.[213]

There is a sulfur supplement called MSM (methylsulfonylmethane) that is widely used to treat arthritis. While sulfur-rich vegetables also contain MSM, they likely contain many other important compounds that work together to assist the functioning of our brain, blood, hair, skin, nails, joints, (head, shoulders, knees, and toes). For this reason, I agree with Dr. Wahls that it is better to get MSM in whole food form by eating sulfur-rich vegetables.[214]

For the purposes of this discussion, sulfur-rich vegetables will include three categories, or families: the cabbage family (or brassica), the garlic and onion family, and the mushroom family. Each of these families have important benefits. While mushrooms are not technically vegetables, it is useful for us to place them in this category. Let's take a look at each of these families.

The Cabbage Family (Brassica)

This family helps to protect our brain cells by promoting the production of glutathione, a hugely important antioxidant that our bodies create out of certain foods.[215] Some foods in this family include broccoli, cauliflower, Brussel sprouts, turnips, rutabaga, radishes, and of course cabbage (all colors). Kale and collards are also in this family, and they overlap with the leafy greens, meaning that you can count them towards either greens or sulfur-rich vegetables (one or the other) in your six to nine fists for the day.[216]

The Garlic and Onion Family

This family includes chives, leeks, shallots, and of course, all types of onions and garlic. Garlic and onions are considered allium vegetables, which are powerful anti-inflammatories and have been studied extensively in their role in cancer prevention.[217, 218] Additionally, aged garlic extract has been shown to reduce dementia and heart-disease risk,[219] but Dr. Wahls points out that other synergistic nutrients of the extract are likely lost during the purification process to make the extracts or isolated nutrients.[220] Rather than supplementing with aged garlic or MSM, we both prefer to get these nutrients in their whole food forms: to eat more garlic, onions, and other allium vegetables.[221] If your healthcare provider advises higher supplementation, however, MSM or aged garlic supplements can be used.[222] You can find more information about these at feedabrain.com/supplements.

The Mushroom Family

Mushrooms are not only an excellent source of sulfur, they also contain a variety of B vitamins as well as other compounds that have been shown to balance the immune system. And a balanced immune system is protective against essentially all chronic health conditions, including autoimmune disease and cancer.[223, 224, 225]

But we should also be aware that mushrooms aren't for everyone. Some individuals may be sensitive to mushrooms and may feel fatigued, brain fog, or headaches after consuming them. If you or your loved one notice negative effects after eating mushrooms, then remove them from the diet, at least temporarily (at least 60 days).

Gastric Feed Information

Because mushrooms aren't for everyone, leave mushrooms out of the diet to remain on the safe side. There are plenty of other sulfur-rich vegetable options, as well as other sources of B vitamins, such as organ meats or some vegan sources like spirulina. You can find this and other alternative supplements for vegans at feedabrain.com/vegan.

TWO TO THREE FISTS OF COLORS

We also want to get our colored vegetables and fruits. Fruits and veggies that are colored throughout, like carrots, beets, berries, kiwis, celery, avocados, etc. are packed with antioxidant power which is very important for our brain health, as well as many other health markers.[226]

Rather than looking at fruits and vegetables separately, we are going to lump them together and separate them by color. Most people aren't aware that avocados, tomatoes, and olives are all fruits anyway. Did you know that cucumbers and zucchinis are technically fruits? The reason it makes sense to separate these plants by color is because the antioxidants and phytonutrients that supply our nervous system are not associated with whether the plant is a fruit or vegetable, but rather *the color* of that fruit or vegetable.[227] When we are talking about this pigment, we do not consider white to be a color, and we are talking about fruits and veggies that are colored all the way through, and not just on the skin.

> **When the deep pigment in a vegetable or fruit is colored all the way through, the concentration of antioxidants is the highest.[228]**

While you are welcome to eat fruits that are not deeply pigmented on the inside and that are only colored on the outside, like apples, bananas, or pears, they do not count towards your two to three fists of colors.[229] Let's not eat them *in place of* all the other foods we want to include in our daily meals.

Antioxidants: What Exactly Do They Do?

Normal metabolism creates a manageable amount of reactive oxygen species (ROS), otherwise known as free radicals. These reactive oxygen species react either with antioxidants or with tissues in the brain and body.[230] When ROS react with tissues in the brain and body, they cause incremental damage. While this is one of the inevitable ways in which we age, antioxidants react with some of the free radicals and reduce their ability to cause damage.[231]

> **Free radicals cause internal damage, but antioxidants can slow that damage down.[232]**

After a concussion/brain injury or throughout a brain disease process, there is a huge increase in the amount of ROS, so we especially want antioxidants to help us to recover.[233] For this reason, it is standard practice for functional neurologists to use extra supplementation of antioxidants and anti-inflammatory compounds to quell the inflammation after a head injury.[234]

As it turns out, the effects of a concussion/brain injury are similar to those of neurodegenerative diseases such as Alzheimer's or Parkinson's.[235] In fact, researchers are looking at TBI as a model for Alzheimer's disease prevention.

At a cellular level, when we look at what happens after a concussion/brain injury, we effectively see the brain age in hyper-speed,[236] and antioxidants help to protect against the effects of aging.

Antioxidants also serve to protect against so much more, including cardiovascular disease, cancer, and dementia.[237]

In addition to these benefits, colored fruits and veggies are especially tasty. There are four different categories that house our colored fruits and veggies: Green, Red, Midnight (purple/blue/black), and Sunset (orange/yellow). "Different colors of vegetables and fruits indicate different properties and different combinations of phytochemicals" that contribute to health.[238]

To me, the most important property of these foods is that they promote healthier brain cell structure and function. They also promote stronger, more elastic blood vessels and improved prostate health.[239] Additionally, they have antibacterial properties, and they protect against DNA damage while supporting immune system, skin, eye, and reproductive health.[240] Deeply pigmented fruits and vegetables promote healthier overall cell structure and function, and remember, *it all comes down to the cell.*

Let's look at some examples of what falls into each of these four categories so that you have an idea of the types of produce to look for.

We want to try to eat several different colors every day.

Green

Unlike leafy greens, which are leaves on a plant, these are the fruits and vegetables which are brightly colored all the way through and not only on the skin. Some examples of green fruits and veggies that are colored throughout include avocados, celery, green peppers, and honey dew melon.

But that's not all. Because of the high antioxidant content of the skins of a few fruits and veggies that are not green throughout, cucumbers with skin, green grapes, and zucchinis are also counted in this group (and are an exception to the general rule that the produce must be deeply pigmented throughout to count as a color).[241]

Red

Some good examples of fruits and veggies that are colored red throughout include beets, blood oranges, radicchio, fresh or frozen red cherries or cranberries (no added sugar), grapefruits, red peppers, raspberries, strawberries, and tomatoes. Like green grapes on the green list, because of the antioxidant content in the skins of red grapes, they count as well.[242]

Midnight (purple/blue/black)

Midnight veggies are pretty rare, but midnight fruits are some of my favorite! Some examples of midnight fruits include blackberries, blueberries, purple figs, and even purple olives (olives are technically a fruit). Again, grapes count here too (black and purple grape).[243]

Sunset (orange/yellow)

Sunset vegetables like golden beets, carrots, squash, pumpkin, sweet potatoes, and orange and yellow peppers are great to roast with sulfur-rich vegetables and then to add to a leafy green salad with plenty of healthy oils and "good fats." Sunset fruits, like oranges, peaches, pineapples, grapefruit, mangoes, and cantaloupe are tasty on their own, or in addition to many dishes.[244]

There is a plethora of delicious fruits and veggies in each of these categories. Again, because different colors indicate different properties and combinations of the phytochemicals that contribute to health, we want to get a variety of colors each day.[245]

The following two handouts are adapted from THE WAHLS PROTOCOL by Terry Wahls and Eve Adamson, copyright ©2014 by Dr. Terry Wahls L.LC. Used by permission of Avery, an imprint of Penguin Publishing Group, a division of Penguin Random House LLC.

*For your convenience, all charts can be found as printable, full-size, color PDF files at feedabrain.com/handouts.

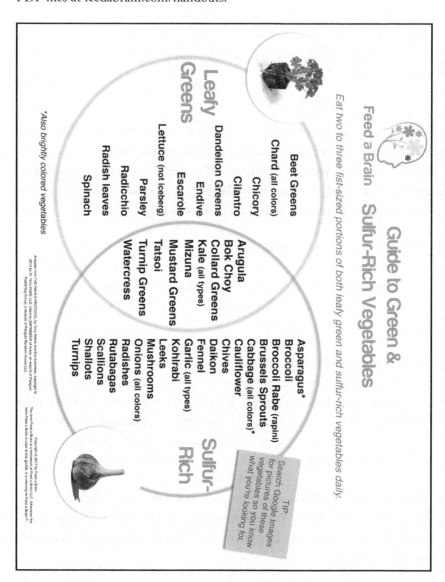

Feed a Brain — Guide to Green & Sulfur-Rich Vegetables

Eat two to three fist-sized portions of both leafy green and sulfur-rich vegetables daily.

Leafy Greens

- Beet Greens
- Chard (all colors)
- Chicory
- Cilantro
- Dandelion Greens
- Endive
- Escarole
- Lettuce (not iceberg)
- Parsley
- Radicchio
- Radish leaves
- Spinach

*Also brightly colored vegetables

- Arugula
- Bok Choy
- Collard Greens
- Kale (all types)
- Mizuna
- Mustard Greens
- Tatsoi
- Turnip Greens
- Watercress

Sulfur-Rich

- Asparagus*
- Broccoli
- Broccoli Rabe (rapini)
- Brussels Sprouts
- Cabbage (all colors)*
- Cauliflower
- Chives
- Daikon
- Fennel
- Garlic (all types)
- Kohlrabi
- Leeks
- Mushrooms
- Onions (all colors)
- Radishes
- Rutabagas
- Scallions
- Shallots
- Turnips

Tip:
Search Google Images for pictures of these vegetables so you know what you're looking for.

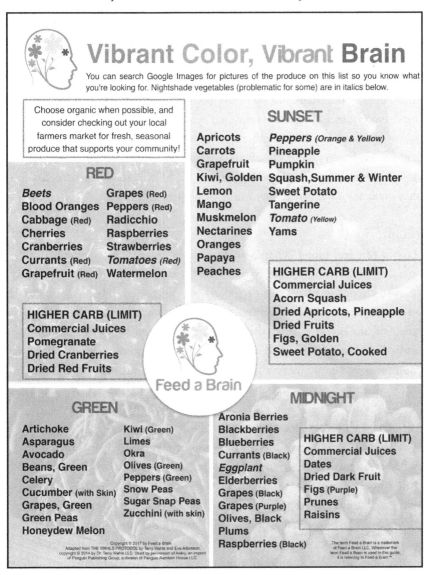

Vibrant Color, Vibrant Brain

You can search Google Images for pictures of the produce on this list so you know what you're looking for. Nightshade vegetables (problematic for some) are in italics below.

Choose organic when possible, and consider checking out your local farmers market for fresh, seasonal produce that supports your community!

RED

Beets	Grapes (Red)
Blood Oranges	Peppers (Red)
Cabbage (Red)	Radicchio
Cherries	Raspberries
Cranberries	Strawberries
Currants (Red)	*Tomatoes* (Red)
Grapefruit (Red)	Watermelon

HIGHER CARB (LIMIT)
Commercial Juices
Pomegranate
Dried Cranberries
Dried Red Fruits

SUNSET

Apricots	*Peppers* (Orange & Yellow)
Carrots	Pineapple
Grapefruit	Pumpkin
Kiwi, Golden	Squash, Summer & Winter
Lemon	Sweet Potato
Mango	Tangerine
Muskmelon	*Tomato* (Yellow)
Nectarines	Yams
Oranges	
Papaya	
Peaches	

HIGHER CARB (LIMIT)
Commercial Juices
Acorn Squash
Dried Apricots, Pineapple
Dried Fruits
Figs, Golden
Sweet Potato, Cooked

Feed a Brain

GREEN

Artichoke	Kiwi (Green)
Asparagus	Limes
Avocado	Okra
Beans, Green	Olives (Green)
Celery	Peppers (Green)
Cucumber (with Skin)	Snow Peas
Grapes, Green	Sugar Snap Peas
Green Peas	Zucchini (with skin)
Honeydew Melon	

MIDNIGHT

Aronia Berries
Blackberries
Blueberries
Currants (Black)
Eggplant
Elderberries
Grapes (Black)
Grapes (Purple)
Olives, Black
Plums
Raspberries (Black)

HIGHER CARB (LIMIT)
Commercial Juices
Dates
Dried Dark Fruit
Figs (Purple)
Prunes
Raisins

Copyright © 2017 by Feed a Brain
Adapted from THE WAHLS PROTOCOL by Terry Wahls and Eve Adamson,
copyright © 2014 by Dr. Terry Wahls LLC. Used by permission of Avery, an imprint
of Penguin Publishing Group, a division of Penguin Random House LLC.

The term Feed a Brain is a trademark of Feed a Brain LLC. Whenever the term Feed a Brain is used in this guide, it is referring to Feed a Brain ™

BALANCING BLOOD SUGAR

The importance of stable blood glucose levels for our brain health cannot be overstated as large fluctuations in blood sugar are a major contributor to neurological damage.[246, 247, 248, 249, 250] Neurodegenerative diseases are much more common among diabetics.[251] In fact, in a 2008 review article published in the *Journal of Diabetes Science and Technology,*researchers call Alzheimer's Disease "Type 3 Diabetes" and this nomenclature is gaining popularity. [252, 253, 254]

When blood sugar is imbalanced, glucose levels in the blood tend to shoot up and down like a roller coaster.[255] Low blood sugar starves the brain of glucose, and neurons can die as a result.[256, 257] When blood sugar is too high, glycation occurs. Glycation is when proteins, which are the most plentiful substances in the brain and body, are bound by sugar.[258] As this occurs, cells are damaged, including brain cells, and aging is accelerated.[259] If you feel tired when you don't eat, notice more energy when you do eat, or if you get irritable when hungry, your blood sugar is probably not stable.[260] This does not necessarily mean you're diabetic, but you may have blood sugar fluctuations that make for a dangerous environment within your brain.

Monitoring

As you can see, blood sugar is an incredibly important biomarker of what stress we are putting on our brain. While it may not be necessary for many of us to check our blood sugar regularly, we don't need to be diabetic to take advantage of this cheap and important tool to monitor our brain health. The levels of our blood glucose throughout the day tell us so much about our brain and overall health, and we have the technology to easily and affordably monitor it by simply using a glucometer. For more information and my preferred glucometer go to feedabrain.com/bloodsugar.

What is a Healthy Blood Sugar Range?

A study using a constant blood sugar monitor measured the normal blood glucose ranges for healthy children, adolescents, and adults aged 9–65. This study found ranges to be between 71–120 mg/dl for 91% of the day with blood glucose very rarely (less than 0.4% of the day) going below 60 mg/dl or over 140 mg/dl.[261] Most functional practitioners agree that a fasting blood sugar, measured first thing in the morning after at least 8 hours without food, should ideally be in the mid- to high-80s, and at least between 85–100 mg/dl.[262] If you find yourself to be off that target and need further support in stabilizing blood sugar, you can find more information and further support at feedabrain.com/bloodsugar.

By including the six to nine fists of fruits and vegetables each day, supplying adequate protein, and removing sugar and processed foods, we are already making important changes that will help to prevent these spikes and dips. Just remember that whenever we eat carbohydrates, we want to eat them with plenty of fat, fiber, and/or protein (or all three), and usually in whole food form.

Eating real food in its whole food form is the most important thing we can do for our brains and bodies.

To keep my own blood sugar stable, I usually start off the day by eating something high in protein and fat within the first two hours after waking. Metabolically, the morning is the worst time to consume a carbohydrate-rich breakfast, yet most of the foods which Americans associate with breakfast are either potentially inflammatory (like yogurt and eggs) or are very high in carbohydrates (like cereal or oatmeal).

Cortisol is a neurohormone which boosts blood sugar,[263] and cortisol levels are highest in the morning. In coupling these high levels of cortisol with a breakfast that is high in carbohydrates, we are setting ourselves up for high blood sugar and an increased risk of developing insulin resistance.[264, 265] So, let's stop having high glycemic or potentially inflammatory foods for breakfast.

Who says we have to eat breakfast foods for breakfast? I like to eat dinner foods for breakfast. I enjoy a "Feed a Brain Breakfast Bowl": some kind of leafy green, mixed with sautéed, roasted, or raw sulfur and colored produce, some sort of delicious meat or fish, and dressed with a whole lot of brain supportive oil. Many mornings I post a picture and the ingredients of my breakfast bowl on Instagram: @feedabrain.

Tips and Tricks to Stabilize Blood Sugar

- Have a breakfast high in fat and protein. I usually have one half to one full fist size piece of some kind of meat with a heavily oiled (good fat) salad that contains all three kinds of produce.
- Eat a little protein and/or good fats every two to three hours.
- Don't eat high-carb foods without fiber, good fat, and/or protein, and keep in mind that grains, even whole grains, are not a good source of fiber, but fruits and vegetables (in their whole food form) are. Some foods which often spike blood sugar and that are usually consumed without fiber, good fat, or protein are sodas (even "diet"), juices, chips, pastries, crackers, and dried fruit. Avoid these foods, especially by themselves.

- Get to sleep before 11 pm, and stop intake of any caffeine after noon. Your adrenals are usually taxed when the sun goes down if you are not sleeping, and the more we tax our adrenals, the more our blood sugar is affected, and our brains are put at risk.
- Only eat whole fruits, not juices.

Don't drink squeezed juices. We want to consume whole fruits. Smoothies have whole fruit. Squeezed juices do not.

When it comes to fruit, we want to try to eat these foods in their whole food form and avoid processed products made with them. Fruit snacks (even sugar free, or "made from 100% juice") are not whole foods, and neither is squeezed juice. When a fruit is squeezed, the juice is collected, the pulp is thrown away, and the fruit is no longer whole. The pulp holds the fiber of the fruit, and without it, we are only getting the sweet liquid by itself. This can very easily spike our blood sugar, negatively impacting our brain.[266]

Fortunately, there are some excellent blenders on the market that make blended juices by vigorously blending produce (in it's whole food form) with water until the produce has a juice-like consistency. These juices do not spike blood sugar like squeezed juice because they contain all the pulp and fiber (remember, fiber, fat, and protein slow the release of sugar into the blood, preventing blood sugar spikes) that is excluded in squeezed juice. You do not need to eliminate squeezed juice from your diet completely, but it should be avoided.

*Also be aware that dried fruit, like raisins, may also spike blood sugar and should also be avoided.

*Lemon and lime juice is not a concern because lemons and limes are lower in sugar and are too sour to consume in large quantities.

Keep Switching it Up

Can you believe our ancestors would have eaten two hundred or more different varieties of plants each year? Today, even if we eat lots of fruits and vegetables, most of us have access to only a handful of different species. There are many different reasons why it is beneficial for us to eat a wide variety of plants, one of these reasons relates to our microbiome, or the beneficial bacteria in our digestive system.

Bacteria are not the enemy of our health as they were once thought to be. In fact, in 2008, the United States National Institutes of Health launched a five-year initiative, with a $115 million budget, to identify and to quantify the microbiome, or "the ecological community of microorganisms that literally share our body space."[267] This initiative sampled both healthy and diseased humans to understand better how this bacterial makeup can either help or harm us.[268]

In late 2013, National Public Radio made an educational and wonderfully understandable video about the microbiome explaining why a favorable population of bacteria living within us promotes health, vitality, and immunity.[269] An unfavorable population, however, may promote the development of disease,[270] and what we eat directly affects this bacterial population.[271] You can find a link to this video at feedabrain.com/microbiome.

Our food is not just food for us. Fibrous plant matter, sugar, and other carbohydrates are also food for our microbiome. Some plants feed one kind of bacteria in our digestive tract while other plants feed other bacterial populations. But, if we eat the same thing every day, one group of bacteria overpowers the other, and our microbiome becomes unbalanced.[272] This can be problematic because different types of bacteria are important for different aspects of our biochemistry.[273] One kind of probiotic, for example, might play a role in blood sugar regulation, another in hunger and weight loss, or another in immunity. If we don't feed many different types of bacteria, certain aspects of our physiology may not function very well.[274]

Another reason why it is beneficial for us to switch up the fruits and vegetables we eat is because most plants have evolved to produce phytochemicals, which are much like thorns on a rose bush, in the sense that they deter animals from eating them, but at a chemical level.[275] At first, by exercising our immune system, these phytochemicals can actually stimulate our cells to function better, but when we eat the same foods every day, the same kinds of phytochemical compounds build up and begin to harm us.[276, 277]

There's a simple solution to this: rotate your produce. Think of it like working out. In the same way that a balanced exercise regimen is much more effective in improving overall strength and performance, a variety of different foods is beneficial to our overall health. If we only do one kind of exercise, we only exercise one group of muscles, and we are prone to injury due to an imbalance of strength. This is like feeding only one group of bacteria that makeup our microbiome while other important bacteria are overrun.

Additionally, the phytochemical buildup that occurs when we eat the same foods, day after day, can become harmful. This is analogous to how doing only one kind of exercise does not give our muscles a chance to recover, and rather than building muscle, we will actually start to harm ourselves.

Let's rotate the produce we eat. For leafy greens, we can eat kale one week, chard the next, then spinach, and then lettuce. For sulfur-rich vegetables, we could eat onions on Monday, broccoli on Wednesday, parsnips on Friday, and cauliflower on Sunday. By rotating the produce we eat, we switch up the compounds that stress us, and we become stronger and healthier.

For this reason, the recipe guidelines provided include several alternative ingredients that still supply the three categories of produce (leafy greens, sulfur, and colors). You can use these recipe guides to rotate the types of produce you consume.

Chapter 7
THE INS — FATS AND NEUROLOGICAL HEALTH

Despite the prevailing nutritional recommendations of the past few decades (which may have guided 60% of Americans to be "overweight," and have likely been large contributors to the fact that the U.S. now consists of about 30% of the world's obese population[278, 279]), several studies demonstrate that saturated animal fats like fatty cuts of meat, butter, and even lard are very beneficial to human health.[280, 281] Because toxins tend to be stored in the fat of animals, it is better to get your fats from clean sources, but don't let the absence of an "organic," "pasture raised," or "grass-fed" label deter you from eating this important nutrient for brain health. I personally eat a lot of grass-fed ghee (clarified butter), and especially while the brain is healing, I encourage you and your loved ones to not avoid animal fats because of their saturated fat content. You can find more information on high-quality ghee and other healthy fats at feedabrain.com/fat.

Over 60% of the weight of the dry matter of the human brain is lipid (fatty acids), and most of these fatty acids are AA (arachidonic acid) and DHA (docosahexaenoic acid).[282] Both of these fatty acids are found in animal fats.

Natural animal fats are brain fuel. High quality, natural, and healthy fat is important brain building nutrition![283, 284, 285]

Our current perception of fat being the number one culprit of poor health in the USA has not only failed to reduce our weight, but this perception has also failed to reduce the number of heart attacks, strokes, cases of diabetes, insulin sensitivity, autism, Alzheimer's, and other mental and chronic diseases.[286]

While most organisms must rely on carbohydrates as their primary fuel source, we humans have actually adapted to be able to metabolize fat.[287] In other words, fat can be used to fuel our brains and bodies when the metabolism has switched from being fueled primarily by glucose (sugar) to being fueled mostly by ketones (fat). Ketones are essentially the breakdown of fats into energy packets that are usable by our brains and bodies.[288] When fat from your food is digested, it enters the blood stream and is filtered through the liver where, when your body is efficient at doing so, the fat is turned into metabolic packets called ketones, which can be used to produce ATP, the energy currency we talked about earlier. [289]

High-quality animal fats and fish oils support the brain and nervous system in many ways. I have mentioned DHA, but there is another fatty acid called EPA that is found in high quality fish and algae oils. EPA works in concert with DHA to reduce inflammation from brain injury or central nervous system disorders, such as stroke and epilepsy.[290, 291] High quality fish oils that contain both EPA and DHA can be found at feedabrain.com/omega.

Learning what fats are healthy to consume can be tricky. Depending on the type, fat can be either an important nutrient to support brain health or it can be harmful. The deciding factors have little to do with whether the fat is saturated or unsaturated. For your convenience, we have created a "Guide to Fats and Oils" handout for you to tack on your fridge and/or to share with your healthcare team.

*For your convenience, all printable charts can be found at: feedabrain.com/handouts.

WHY ARE HUMANS ABLE TO METABOLIZE FAT?

The reason that humans have adapted to metabolize in this manner may have been to survive arctic climates that do not have vegetation year round. Healthy human metabolism should be able to switch from fat burning to sugar burning depending on the foods available. When early humans were in an arctic climate in the winter, sugar and carbs were scarce so their metabolism adapted to be primarily fat burning.[292] Think about Eskimo groups like the Inuit, whose diet consisted mostly of a variety of fish, seals, whales and caribou. When these cultures did not have vegetation-like plants and grains to fuel them through the winter, their primary fuel source became fat. Alternatively to the metabolism of humans in a vegetation-scarce climate, when early humans were in a tropical climate in the summer, fat was scarce, so their metabolism adapted to be primarily sugar burning.[293] Today, because the prevalent nutritional guidelines have been primarily promoting carbohydrates, most of us have a metabolism that is set to be primarily sugar burning.

WHY SHOULD WE EAT FAT?

One of the reasons why we should use this alternate fuel source is for better brain health. Ketogenic metabolism has protective effects on the brain in general,[294] and can even be used therapeutically as a treatment for epilepsy and neurodegenerative disorders including Alzheimer's[295] and Parkinson's[296] disease. My favorite finding is that this kind of metabolism has also been shown to be therapeutic after traumatic brain injury and stroke.[297, 298, 299, 300, 301]

Unfortunately, most of us are not used to breaking down fat because we tend to consume plenty of carbs and sugars so that ketogenic metabolism is not necessary and is therefore not triggered. Switching metabolism from primarily glucose (sugar burner) to primarily ketones (fat burner) can be very uncomfortable and bring on intense cravings for sugar and carbs like pasta, bread, desserts, donuts, cookies, or candies for some time while ketones are being created in the liver and this new fuel source is adopted. So how can we switch metabolism when our liver is not used to breaking down fat?

SWITCHING TO KETOGENIC METABOLISM

Luckily, there is a way to avoid these cravings for sugar and carbohydrates, and to smooth out this transition while eating according to this meal plan. The most effective method to experience a much smoother transition is to introduce exogenous ketones to deliver the fuel of fat right away.

What Are Exogenous Ketones?

Now that we know what ketones are, what does "exogenous" mean? When ketones are created in the liver, we refer to them as endogenous. Let's breakdown what "endogenous" and "exogenous" mean. The prefix "endo" means inside, where "exo" means outside. In this case we are talking about inside or outside of the body. The latin word "geno" means to give birth to or to create. This means that something that is created in our bodies can be called endogenous where something created outside of our bodies is called exogenous.

If our body is not adapted to create endogenous ketones and we begin a high fat/low carbohydrate diet, we often enter an uncomfortable period (otherwise known as the "keto flu") where we experience ravenous cravings for sugar and carbohydrates.[302] To prevent this uncomfortable period while providing this neuroprotective fuel source, we can introduce exogenous ketones while introducing the high fat and low carbohydrate foods outlined in this guide.[303] In doing so, we will encourage our liver to adapt to this neuroprotective fuel source.[304] Try starting everyday with some exogenous ketones in conjunction with a high fat breakfast. For more information and links to where you can find quality exogenous ketones, go to feedabrain.com/keto.

FAT GUIDELINES
We need fat, but we need the right kind, and again, it's not about saturated vs. unsaturated fat. For the promotion of health, we want to follow a few guidelines and understand a few concepts pertaining to fat.

- *Fat Guideline 1: Liberally consume fats from sustainably raised animals and wild caught fish.*

Humans have been liberally consuming healthy fats like animal fats for hundreds of thousands of years. Saturated animal fat from healthy animals is not the major player that makes people fat. Several studies show that saturated fat intake is not linked to heart disease, stroke, type 2 diabetes or dying of any cause.[305, 306, 307] In fact, the dietary perspective that saturated fat is bad for our health is finally beginning to change, with *Time Magazine* recently publishing an article titled: "Ending The War on Fat"[308] explaining how and why we were wrong in attempting to promote health by avoiding all saturated fats.

- *Fat Guideline 2: Avoid or eliminate hydrogenated and partially hydrogenated oils as well as artificial trans fats.*

While the science on saturated fat has been skewed, it is well documented and accepted that hydrogenated oils and artificial trans fats have adverse health effects, including detrimental effects to the brain.[309, 310] While it is required

60

that trans fats above 1g per serving be labeled in the United States, many scientists and citizens alike believe that ANY amount should be labeled, or better yet, that all artificial trans fat be completely banned from the food supply.[311]

- *Fat Guideline 3: Avoid industrial seed oils, like canola oil and vegetable oil.*

Our ancestors did not evolve using massive machines to squeeze hundreds of thousands of seeds in order to extract the oil to fry something or to drizzle on a salad. These seed and vegetable oils were not available before the industrial revolution, which makes them a very new addition to the human diet. The heavy duty machinery that is required to extract these oils is the reason they are often referred to as "industrial seed oils," and they are often even deodorized to mask that they are spoiled through oxidation.[312]

- *Fat Guideline 4: Liberally consume cold pressed oils from fruits that have large seeds (olive oil, avocado oil, coconut oil, etc.).*

Cold pressed fruit oils with large seeds have been used since the biblical times, and they are well studied.[313] Some of the health benefits of cold pressed olive oil,[314] avocado oil,[315] and coconut oil[316] range from cardiovascular to antioxidant to neurological benefits.

What is Oil Oxidation? Oil oxidation is a process that degrades the quality of an oil, rendering it unhealthy. In fact, oxidized oils are considered cytotoxic, or toxic to living cells, and genotoxic, or toxic to our DNA.[317] Oxidized oils, even if they were once considered healthy, are no longer able to supply the brain with good functional lipids (fats). These oils also produce cellular damage in the heart, liver, kidney, and brain.[318] Oxidized oils contribute to overall oxidative stress, producing even more reactive oxygen species, which we talked about earlier (in the "Antioxidants: What exactly do they do?" section of the book).[319]

Oils are sometimes obviously oxidized, like when an oil tastes or smells rancid, but oxidation also occurs in ways that we cannot easily detect. Oxidation most frequently occurs when oils are heated past their smoke point temperature. When this occurs, we may see or smell smoke, but not always. Almost every oil that is used for deep frying is likely heated past its smoke point temperature and is therefore oxidized, so fried foods should also be avoided (unless fried in avocado oil or another oil with a high smoke point temperature).[320, 321] Worse still, many industrial seed oils are heated to high temperatures and are oxidized and then deodorized before they are even bottled.[322] This is yet another reason to avoid them.

The brain requires healthy fats to function well and replacing those functional fats with less functional fats, such as artificial trans fats, industrial seed oils, and oxidized oils can hinder our brain function. Some fats are very healthy and functional before they are oxidized, but they have such a low smoke point temperature that they are not to be used for cooking. Some examples of these oils include fish oils, MCT oil, and cocoa butter.

- *Fat Guideline 5: Avoid fats that have been heated past their smoke point.*

Good fats are very good for the brain, but they are not to be heated past their smoke points. Below is a guide that will help you to determine which oils support brain health, which do not, and which oils are best for different kinds of cooking. I especially like to cook with grass-fed ghee (clarified butter) and avocado oil (similar to olive oil, but with a much higher smoke point). Olive oil oxidizes at a lower temperature than both of these, but as long as we're not heating it past 375°F (190°C), it is a perfectly acceptable cooking oil for medium/low heat. Refer to the guide below:

*For your convenience, all printable charts can be found at: feedabrain.com/handouts.

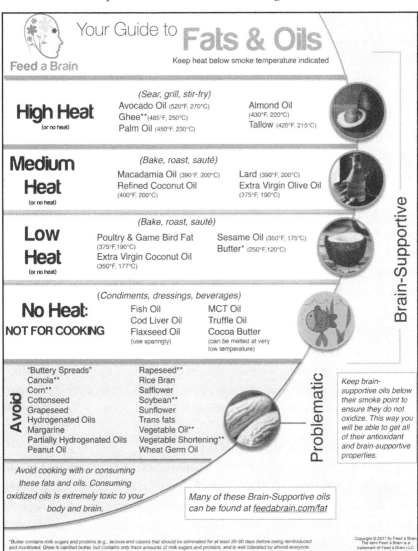

Your Guide to **Fats & Oils**

Feed a Brain — Keep heat below smoke temperature indicated

High Heat (or no heat)
(Sear, grill, stir-fry)
Avocado Oil (520°F, 270°C)
Ghee** (485°F, 250°C)
Palm Oil (450°F, 230°C)
Almond Oil (430°F, 220°C)
Tallow (420°F, 215°C)

Medium Heat (or no heat)
(Bake, roast, sauté)
Macadamia Oil (390°F, 200°C)
Refined Coconut Oil (400°F, 200°C)
Lard (390°F, 200°C)
Extra Virgin Olive Oil (375°F, 190°C)

Low Heat (or no heat)
(Bake, roast, sauté)
Poultry & Game Bird Fat (375°F,190°C)
Extra Virgin Coconut Oil (350°F, 177°C)
Sesame Oil (350°F, 175°C)
Butter* (250°F,120°C)

No Heat:
NOT FOR COOKING
(Condiments, dressings, beverages)
Fish Oil
Cod Liver Oil
Flaxseed Oil
(use sparingly)
MCT Oil
Truffle Oil
Cocoa Butter
(can be melted at very low temperature)

Avoid
"Buttery Spreads"
Canola**
Corn**
Cottonseed
Grapeseed
Hydrogenated Oils
Margarine
Partially Hydrogenated Oils
Peanut Oil
Rapeseed**
Rice Bran
Safflower
Soybean**
Sunflower
Trans fats
Vegetable Oil**
Vegetable Shortening**
Wheat Germ Oil

Avoid cooking with or consuming these fats and oils. Consuming oxidized oils is extremely toxic to your body and brain.

Brain-Supportive

Problematic

Keep brain-supportive oils below their smoke point to ensure they do not oxidize. This way you will be able to get all of their antioxidant and brain-supportive properties.

Many of these Brain-Supportive oils can be found at feedabrain.com/fat

Butter contains milk sugars and proteins (e.g., lactose and casein) that should be eliminated for at least 30-90 days before being reintroduced and monitored. Ghee is clarified butter, but contains only trace amounts of milk sugars and proteins, and is well tolerated by almost everyone.

WHAT ABOUT CALORIES?

There is so much attention on counting calories, but what exactly are they? Calories are actually a measure of potential energy or the measurement of how much energy could possibly be utilized in a food. Food is important in fueling our brain and bodies, and calories are a measurement of that fuel. Many often talk of calories as a bad thing, but it has become very clear to me that the term "calories" is an over generalized marker. There are good calories and bad calories.[323] Some calories don't serve us, and some do.

Good Calories vs. Bad Calories

- Bad calories are foods that provide energy (calories) but contain little nutrient value. The two main examples that I would consider "bad calories" are sugar and flour (even gluten free).
- Good calories are nutrient rich foods that also supply energy.

Limit bad calories and eat a lot of good calories. We want the foods that we eat to be very rich in nutrients, and because good fats are so important for our brain health, the energy that we get from these fats are "good calories."

I consider animal fats and cold pressed seed oils (not heated past their smoke point) to be good calories, especially when those animals are sustainably raised. For numerous reasons, which I will expand upon in this chapter, I have come to understand that diets rich in natural fats and oils can be excellent for brain and body health.

The idea of more calories consumed than calories burned as a contributor to weight gain and disease has been shown to not always be the case. Studies of high-fat diets showing weight *loss* especially debunk this over generalization.[324, 325] I perceive food as a substance that will either serve me or not, even if that food is high in calories or fat.

WHAT ABOUT CHOLESTEROL?

Soon after my brain injury, I showed what my functional neurologist would consider low cholesterol on a blood panel, and as far as I was concerned at the time, this was good news. The doctors at the hospital were also not concerned about this, as Mayo Clinic (at the time of this writing) says that any level of total cholesterol below 200 mg/dL is "desirable."[326] Does this mean that absolutely no cholesterol would be healthy? What is the function of cholesterol? Does it cause heart disease, and do humans need it?

Almost every time that I advocate traditional animal fats as being important brain nutrition, for everything from brain injury rehabilitation to the neuroprotective effects that prevent seizures,[327] a concern is brought up about cholesterol. And with the scary prevailing thoughts about the dangers of cholesterol and heart disease, it is no wonder that it is a topic of concern. People have been told that foods like eggs, bacon, and saturated fats from meat and butter raise our cholesterol levels, and that high cholesterol clogs our arteries and gives us heart attacks. This idea is so deeply ingrained within our culture that very few even question it. Let's clarify what cholesterol is, what HDL and LDL are, and whether cholesterol is the *cause* of heart disease or whether it is just a marker. If you already understand that cholesterol is not something that needs to be avoided, feel free to skip to the end of this chapter.

When exploring research, a very important concept is that correlation does not imply causation, meaning that just because two things always occur together does not necessarily show us that one causes the other. For example, fire trucks tend to congregate wherever there is a fire, but of course, the fire trucks are not necessarily the *cause* of the fire. While cholesterol might be a *marker* for heart disease, it is not necessarily the *cause* of heart disease.

Can My Cholesterol Be Too Low?

A deficiency in cholesterol is found in a congenital condition, or a condition that one is born with, known as Smith-Lemli-Opitz syndrome (SLOS).[328] Most conceptions with SLOS do not live to reach birth, which is strong evidence that cholesterol is essential to fertility and the life and growth of a human being. In the rare cases where this child is not spontaneously aborted, the child is born with a plethora of facial and skeletal abnormalities, as well as mental problems like autism, hyperactivity, and attention deficit disorders, as well as self-injurious, aggressive behavior, and even mental retardation.[329] This child may also suffer from endocrine dysfunction and serious digestive problems. The usual treatment for this syndrome has been a diet rich in cream and egg yolks, which are rich in naturally occurring cholesterol.[330]

Lowered cholesterol from statin use is also associated with mood disorders and depression.[331] Deficiency of cholesterol also affects the release of neurotransmitters in the brain and adversely impacts cognition.[332]

As we can see, cholesterol is very important for human growth and development, so what exactly does cholesterol do for adults?

What is the Function of Cholesterol?

Cholesterol is part of what makes up the outer membrane of every cell within an animal body.[333] This membrane is also known as the lipid bilayer and it is one of the most important parts of every animal cell.[334] Cholesterol is also found at the synapse between every axon and dendrite within the brain.[335] This is where communication between neurons allows the brain to direct everything that we do, say, or think. This means that cholesterol is needed for neurons within the brain to communicate effectively, and that cholesterol plays an important role in synaptogenesis, or the building of new connections among neurons (connections which are especially important after a brain injury).[336, 337] Cholesterol is even important in digestion and is the precursor to, or the building blocks that are used to make, sex hormones such as estrogen and testosterone.[338, 339]

What Exactly Are HDL and LDL?

Most people are under the impression that there is good cholesterol and bad cholesterol, referring to HDL as the "good cholesterol" and LDL as the "bad cholesterol," but what are HDL and LDL? HDL and LDL are actually acronyms for high density and low-density lipoproteins.[340] Lipoproteins are not cholesterol, but the transporters or carriers of lipid bioactive factors, or materials that have a significant biochemical function (like cholesterol).[341] In other words, lipoproteins carry materials that are vitally important to life, and as it turns out, cholesterol is one of these vitally important bioactive factors.[342]

How and Why Does Cholesterol Clog Arteries?

What has been found in clogged arteries is almost always a build up of certain kinds of LDL particles within the blood while inflammation is present.[343] C-reactive protein, or CRP, is a protein found in the blood, the levels of which have been shown to rise in response to inflammation.[344] Thus, CRP is a good indicator of inflammation. Interestingly, CRP shows a stronger correlation to heart disease than LDL cholesterol levels.[345] And even more notably, in most healthy individuals, an increase in the consumption of dietary cholesterol does not seem to increase serum cholesterol, or cholesterol in the blood.[346]

Without inflammation, cholesterol is usually able to move freely within the blood and not clog arteries, just as it moves throughout the blood everywhere else where there is no clot. But the prevailing understanding is that if the cholesterol wasn't there, there would be no clogged arteries. While this may be true, the inflammation should be the focus of changes. If dietary cholesterol is cut, it sets off a stress response in the body that can lead to excess production of cholesterol,[347] or there may also be other problems associated with a cholesterol deficiency, like all the devastating conditions of SLOS.

As Dr. David Perlmutter states, it is carbs — not cholesterol — that cause high cholesterol.[348] Our bodies truly need cholesterol from dietary sources for optimal brain function.[349]

Clogged Arteries: Traffic Jams

I like to think of arteries as a wide highway with six or seven lanes in which semi-trucks transport goods to different locations in the body. Think of the semi-trucks as lipoproteins and the goods that these semi-trucks transport as cholesterol and other important bioactive factors. If all but one lane has closed on this highway, there is a traffic jam or a clogged artery. We have two choices: we can decrease the number of trucks (by taking statins), but then supplies do not get to their destinations, or alternatively, we can fix the road.

A statin drug does not address the cause of the lane closures (inflammation), but simply decreases the number of semi-trucks (lipoproteins transporting cholesterol). Additionally, because cholesterol is required to build and maintain cell membranes, not having enough cholesterol means that there are not enough supplies for new cells to generate and function. We need to fix the road by decreasing the inflammation in the body.

For me, a low functional level of cholesterol meant that I was not providing the supplies to build new neurons or synapses within my brain and the work I was doing through therapy was not being nutritionally supported. After beginning a higher saturated fat and cholesterol diet, in conjunction with other nutritional practices (most of which are covered in this guide), I began to regain clarity, and I started to write my blog (adventuresinbraininjury.com).

Now that we are over our fat phobia, I'd like to share a morning beverage with you that includes a fair amount of fat for neuroprotection, and is a perfect addition to a "Feed a Brain Breakfast Bowl." This recipe also supplies turmeric and black pepper, which have been shown to greatly reduce inflammation in the brain when taken together.[350, 351] This and other recipes can be found at feedabrain.com/recipes. We'll be posting fresh recipes as we develop them!

GOLDEN GLOBE LATTE

Servings 2

Ingredients:
- 1 can full-fat coconut milk, bone broth, or water
- 1 tsp turmeric
- ½ tsp cinnamon
- 1 tsp - 1 tbsp. of ghee
- 1 tsp - 1 tbsp. of coconut oil
- 1 pinch of black pepper (increases bioavailability of turmeric)
- ½ fist sized piece of fresh or frozen peach, or other golden colored fruit like cantaloupe, mango, pineapple, etc.
- Optional – 1 scoop of exogenous ketones (feedabrain.com/keto)
- Optional - ¼ of a fist-sized avocado
- Optional - 1 pinch of cayenne pepper (for extra heat)

Instructions:
1. Pour coconut milk, broth, or water into a small saucepan and heat over medium until hot but not boiling.
2. While liquid is heating, assemble all other ingredients in a blender or a stick blending container.
3. When liquid is hot, add to other ingredients and blend until smooth.
4. Garnish with a sprinkle of cinnamon and enjoy!

Chapter 8
THE INS — HYDRATION AND MACRONUTRIENTS

HYDRATION

For any of the benefits that we have talked about so far to be effective, it is very important for us to be sure to supply adequate hydration. We are all aware that we need to be hydrated to live, but another very important function of hydration is to help us to move toxins out of our bodies, so we want to supply more than just enough to survive.

The amount of water that we consider to be optimal is dependent on many factors including how much water is in the foods we eat. If we are supplying nutrition via a gastric tube, we may want to work with a qualified healthcare professional to determine this amount, but for healthy adults, we can generally divide our weight in pounds by two, and use that number to determine how many ounces of water to drink each day as a minimum requirement.[352]

So if you weigh about 160 pounds (like me), you would divide that number by two and know to drink at least 80 ounces of water. Using a different method of measurement, since there are about 30 ounces in a liter, and about 2 pounds in a kilogram, we can divide our weight in kilograms by 30 to determine how many liters to drink.

If you weigh about 72.5 kilograms (like me), you would divide that number by 30 and know to drink at least 2.4 liters of water a day. Again, this amount is a guideline for a minimum requirement. I tend to drink much more than my minimum requirement of 80 ounces and consume more like 140 ounces of water per day. This converts to about 4 liters per day which is far more than my required 2.4 liters.

It is important that we do not supply too much or too little water (over hydrate or under hydrate); yet, there is quite a bit of wiggle room for us. I absolutely love a certain water bottle that is entirely spill proof and doesn't need to have the top opened in order to drink from it. Because the bottle is itself so convenient, I end up drinking more water. A simple purchase like that can ensure we are properly hydrated and improve our health dramatically. You can see this product and more information about hydration at feedabrain.com/hydration.

For nurses and dietitians, there is a good article concerning hydration management that was published in *Nursing Times:* "Maintaining hydration in enteral tube feeding." You can find this article, and other important information at feedabrain.com/hydration.

*Keep in mind that needs may increase based on physical activity, climate, or other medical needs, so work with a qualified healthcare provider.
* Depending on the amount of salt, bone broth may also count towards your hydration, meaning that a cup of unsalted broth can potentially be counted as a cup of water.
* Bone broth contains protein as well.

MACRONUTRIENTS
Macronutrients are broken down into three main categories: carbohydrates, proteins, and fats.[353] While most of us can rely on our appetite to guide our protein requirements, these requirements can vary significantly depending on the stage of recovery. Additionally, a patient may be unable to communicate or could potentially have damaged areas to his/her brain that affect appetite. Work with your dietitian to determine requirements, especially for patients who cannot communicate or perceive their appetite. Again, my desire to help is immense. To help navigate these issues, I offer one-on-one consultations at feedabrain.com/consult and we are also working on courses and other resources that will be offered at feedabrain.com/education.

This book will provide some general guidelines and formulas that can be used to estimate amounts of required macronutrients, but keep in mind that these are only estimates of average needs for a healthy individual, and those in critical care can rarely be considered to have a "normal" metabolism.

Jeremy Lampel, MS, RD, CDE has shared with us a handout which he uses to inform his patients of how the macronutrients of their diets might be distributed for different conditions. It is advised that you bring these guidelines to your dietitian or other qualified healthcare provider.

*For your convenience, all charts can be found as printable, full-size, color PDF files at feedabrain.com/handouts.

Macronutrient Ratios

Health conditions, age, gender, and lifestyle determine how much of each macronutrient should be consumed per day. The Ketogenic and Low Carb ratios provided below are typically appropriate for neurological conditions. The amounts (provided in grams) are guidelines for healthy average size men and women.

Carbohydrates

	% Carbs	Carb (Grams) for Men (2600 kcal/day)	Carb (Grams) for Women (2000 kcal diet)	Goal/Population
Ketogenic	< 10%	< 65 g	< 50 g	- Epilepsy, brain injury or neurodegenerative disease (Parkinson's, Alzheimer's, etc.) - Severe blood sugar problems
Low Carb	10 – 15%	65 – 100 g	50 – 75 g	- Weight loss - Blood sugar regulation - Mood disturbances - Blood sugar regulation - Digestive problems
Moderate Carb	15 – 40%	100 – 200 g	75 – 150 g	- Generally healthy - Maintain weight - Adrenal fatigue - Maintain weight - Adrenal fatigue - Hypothyroidism - Familial Hypercholesterolemia
High Carb	> 40%	> 200 g	> 150 g	- Athletes and highly active people - Trying to gain weight/muscle - Fast metabolism - Pregnant/breastfeeding

Fat

Once you've determined your carb and protein levels, the rest of your calories will come from fat. This could be as high as 80-85% fat on a ketogenic/low carbohydrate/low protein diet.

Protein

Goal/Population	% Protein	Protein (Grams) for Men (2600 kcal diet)	Protein (Grams) for Women (2000 kcal diet)
Generally healthy or pregnant	10 – 20%	65 – 130 g	50 – 100 g
Weight loss, blood, sugar problems, adding muscle mass	20 – 35%	130 – 230 g	100 – 176 g

Jeremy Lampel MS RD CDE |

PROTEIN

Dr. Terry Wahls says that adults need at least 6 ounces (170 grams) of animal meat per day, and preferably closer to 12 ounces (340 grams), but up to twenty-one ounces (595 grams) per day.[354] General macronutrient guidelines tend to be measured as grams of the macronutrient protein, but not grams of a protein containing food like meat. An 8 ounces serving of beef, for example, weighs about 227 grams, but it only contains 61 grams of actual protein. This becomes confusing when measuring actual food, so we might instead use this guideline as a ballpark: 0.06 - 0.09 ounces of meat per pound of body weight (3.69 grams - 5.67 grams of meat per kilogram of body weight).

So if you, like me, weigh about 160 pounds (about 72 kilograms), then we aim for 9.6 ounces - 14.4 ounces (272 grams - 408 grams) of meat per day. But what does that look like? Let's simplify even further and measure using the size of our fists. The size of my hand formed into a closed fist is close to the size of a 6-8 ounce steak (170-227 grams). So this is the guideline that I like to use:

We want to eat more than one, but up to three fist-sized pieces of meat per day.

You may use these formulas as a ballpark, but again, we encourage you to work with a dietitian, nutritionist, or physician.

CARBOHYDRATES

Now that we can see how much produce we want to be eating, let's strategize how we are going to supply these foods every day. Some of us may be able to get pre-made meals from feedabrain.com/premade, or we can prepare our food ahead of time to get the benefits of convenience combined with excellent nutrition. Batch cooking, meal prep, or bulk cooking is when we prepare most or all of our meals and snacks for the entire week on one day.

We are all very busy with so many things in our lives that food can move way down on our priority list, especially in the face of difficulty. With our busy schedules, we often end up eating a lot of foods that we should have little room for when eating the six to nine fists of brain building produce. But the information contained in this book should really bring the power of the right kind of nutrition to the forefront. Brain nutrition is made so much easier by having meals organized and ready-made, and batch cooking can actually be a fun family activity!

Throughout the beginning stages of changing my diet, when I was hungry (which was almost always), I was incredibly tempted to eat whatever was available at that moment. My mother and I were dealing with immense pressure, pain, loss, and other stressors. We had far too much happening to be able to cook each meal, let alone to think about what those meals might be. As we became more in touch with the healing power of the right nutrition, it became clear that we needed to have these brain-healing foods on hand.

Getting These Nutrients Realistically

My mother and I would batch cook on Sunday when I didn't have therapy. We would go shopping and get roughly equal amounts of sulfur-rich and colored produce for roasting. Some of my favorite colored and sulfur-rich produce for roasting are listed in the Batch Cooking Handout on the next page.

My mother and I would then chop these into roughly inch-size cubes or similar sized pieces or slices. These would be arranged in a large, oven-safe roasting pan. We would add a healthy oil with a smoke point higher than 350°F (232°C), like avocado or olive oil, salt and pepper to taste, and then roast for 30-60 minutes. Afterward, we would pack these roasted veggies in Tupperware and store them in the fridge.

*For your convenience, all charts can be found as printable, full-size, color PDF files at feedabrain.com/handouts.

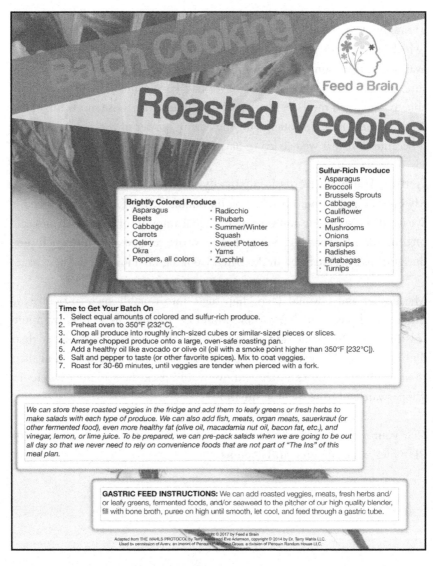

Roasted Veggies

Feed a Brain

Brightly Colored Produce
- Asparagus
- Beets
- Cabbage
- Carrots
- Celery
- Okra
- Peppers, all colors
- Radicchio
- Rhubarb
- Summer/Winter Squash
- Sweet Potatoes
- Yams
- Zucchini

Sulfur-Rich Produce
- Asparagus
- Broccoli
- Brussels Sprouts
- Cabbage
- Cauliflower
- Garlic
- Mushrooms
- Onions
- Parsnips
- Radishes
- Rutabagas
- Turnips

Time to Get Your Batch On
1. Select equal amounts of colored and sulfur-rich produce.
2. Preheat oven to 350°F (232°C).
3. Chop all produce into roughly inch-sized cubes or similar-sized pieces or slices.
4. Arrange chopped produce onto a large, oven-safe roasting pan.
5. Add a healthy oil like avocado or olive oil (oil with a smoke point higher than 350°F [232°C]).
6. Salt and pepper to taste (or other favorite spices). Mix to coat veggies.
7. Roast for 30-60 minutes, until veggies are tender when pierced with a fork.

We can store these roasted veggies in the fridge and add them to leafy greens or fresh herbs to make salads with each type of produce. We can also add fish, meats, organ meats, sauerkraut (or other fermented food), even more healthy fat (olive oil, macadamia nut oil, bacon fat, etc.), and vinegar, lemon, or lime juice. To be prepared, we can pre-pack salads when we are going to be out all day so that we never need to rely on convenience foods that are not part of "The Ins" of this meal plan.

GASTRIC FEED INSTRUCTIONS: We can add roasted veggies, meats, fresh herbs and/or leafy greens, fermented foods, and/or seaweed to the pitcher of our high quality blender, fill with bone broth, puree on high until smooth, let cool, and feed through a gastric tube.

Adapted from THE WAHLS PROTOCOL by Terry Wahls and Eve Adamson, copyright ©2014 by Dr. Terry Wahls L.LC. Used by permission of Avery, an imprint of Penguin Publishing Group, a division of Penguin Random House LLC.

With these veggies, I could easily and accessibly have brain-building food at any point by simply adding them to leafy greens to make a salad. My mother and I would get a large container of pre-washed mixed greens, spinach, or arugula, so leafy greens were always readily available. When making salads, I could add these roasted veggies along with meats, sauerkraut or other fermented foods, and even healthy fat like olive oil, macadamia nut oil, or almond oil (smoke point is not important when we are not heating the oil). My mother and I tried to always pre-pack salads when we would be out all day so that I would never need to rely on convenience foods that were not part of "The Ins" of this meal plan. I would even throw these roasted veggies into a bowl with some bone broth, and then add meats, fresh herbs (cilantro, basil, or parsley) and/or greens, and spices. This made for several possibilities for soups that contained so many of the ingredients our brains crave.

By always having brain-building foods on hand, any reservations that I had towards preparing these meals began to fade. Once we became accustomed to making a small time commitment and gathering the foods we needed in a single trip, we were able to manage the other important aspects of recovery without the added stress of finding the foods that would benefit our efforts.

It was admittedly tricky to find these vegetables at first. I had never knowingly tried some of them. After becoming familiar with some of these ingredients, the act of cutting them up, roasting them, and then packing them into containers was completely worthwhile. I now had a reliable strategy to supply the nutrients needed to rebuild the connections in my brain.

Gastric Feed Information

We can use these batch-cooked veggies to create soups that may be blended in a high-quality blender (like a Blendtec™ or Vitamix™) to make purees for gastric feeding. Add roasted veggies, meats, fresh herbs, healthy fats, and leafy greens to the blender pitcher, fill with bone broth, puree on high until smooth, let cool, and feed through a gastric tube. (See the Gastric Tube Feed Creation Instructions (available at feedabrain.com/handouts).

FATS

This section is going to be short because there is no real hard and fast measurement for the amount of fat that this meal plan outlines. Instead, we can stay within the carb and protein levels outlined and get the rest of our calories from the good fats outlined. This could make our fat consumption as high as 80-85% of calories on a ketogenic/low carbohydrate/low-moderate protein diet (see the Macronutrient Ratios Handout). The Feed a Brain guidelines are certainly "fat forward," or "pro fat," so don't be shy with your intake of the brain supportive fats and oils. (See the Guide to Fats and Oils handout). As an example of the quantity of fat I like to get, in addition to a salad with all three types of produce, plenty of meat, and at least a tablespoon of a brain supportive oil, I also often start my day with a morning beverage that contains at least a tablespoon of brain supportive fat like ghee. The Golden Globe Latte Recipe in this book is an example of one of these fat-forward morning beverages. If you do well with coffee in the morning (I usually don't), make your coffee with butter (if well tolerated), ghee, coconut oil, MCT oil, or other brain supportive fats, which can all be found at feedabrain.com/fat. Doing so is a very appropriate addition to a high protein/low carb breakfast.

Chapter 9
THE INS — NUTRIENTS FOR SYNAPTOGENESIS

Synaptogenesis occurs when neurons grow and connect with each other. This is one of the mechanisms by which the brain builds and repairs itself, so synaptogenesis is especially important after a concussion/brain injury.[355] Synaptogenesis is essentially the creation of connections in the brain which create our habits. As we all know, there are good habits and bad habits. If we practice doing something the wrong way, we strengthen a pathway to do that thing the wrong way. This is known as negative plasticity.[356] Synaptogenesis is something we want to support, but it is also very important that we stimulate our brains in a desirable way, like through targeted therapy, positivity, mindfulness, and meditation, so that we don't create undesirable neuronal connections like bad habits or negative thought patterns.[357]

Coming back to the analogy I borrowed from Dr. Alex Vasquez, DC, ND, DO, FACN, let's again think of neurons as plants, and the cells that support neurons (glia) as the soil that the plants are potted in. If a plant is wilting and dying, it does not take a scientist with a degree in botany to nurse the wilting plant back to health. It takes someone with a "green thumb" to provide good soil, water, sunlight, and a little encouragement (therapy). If we can support the environment that the plants are potted in then we can begin to rebuild some of the damaged connections within the brain and restore the functionality and communication between neurons. In other words, the neurons of the nervous system are designed to heal themselves, as long as they are given the right ingredients and the right environment to do so. And what is really exciting is that we can nutritionally affect the glia to be the healthiest soil it can be so that it can support and maintain the functions of neurons, as well as ensure a constant supply of nutrients.

The work of Dr. Richard Wurtman MD, a Distinguished Professor of Neuroscience in MIT's Department of Brain & Cognitive Sciences, shows us the importance of specific nutrients in the developing and recovering brain. In many of his articles, including this one published in the 2009 *Annual Review of Nutrition,* from MIT's Department of Brain & cognitive Sciences, titled "Use of Phosphatide Precursors to Promote Synaptogenesis,"[358] three key nutrients are described to support the membranes needed for making these connections. He has since published more articles describing these nutrients and their effect on aging, diseased, and injured brains.[359, 360, 361, 362]

These three nutrients are:
- Choline, an essential nutrient that is used in the synthesis of components in cell membranes.
- Docosahexaenoic acid (DHA), an Omega-3 polyunsaturated fatty acid.
- Uridine, one of the five nucleotides that make our DNA and RNA.

While infants get all three of these nutrients from mother's milk, Dr. Wurtman says that there is no food or combination of foods that we adults typically consume to significantly increase blood levels of all three key ingredients.[363] He specifically points out that increasing uridine in the blood is nearly impossible without supplementation or human mother's milk.[364] Because I agree with Dr. Wahls that there are likely synergistic compounds in foods, I like to supplement all three of these nutrients in addition to eating the foods that supply each of them, even if they may not increase that particular nutrient in the blood. Let's explore what these nutrients are and the foods where they can be found, and then we will talk about supplementation and how we can supply these in gastric feeds. You can find these synaptogenic supplements at feedabrain.com/synapto.

CHOLINE

Choline is an essential nutrient that is found in high concentrations in sources like meat (especially organ meats), fish, and egg yolks. There is also some choline found in cauliflower, broccoli, collard greens, beans (not encouraged), and soy milk (not advised) as well. Choline is very important for building and maintaining the cell and neuronal membranes of the brain and body. [365]

It is also essential in making acetylcholine, a neurotransmitter that is associated with memory and movement. Acetylcholine is the most common neurotransmitter in our bodies. It has very important functions in both the autonomic nervous system and digestion, as well as muscle control and strength.[366] In the brain, it plays a large role in arousal, attention, and motivation.[367]

Supplementation Information

Citicoline, a good supplemental form of choline, has been shown to not only enhance memory[368] but also to reduce brain edema (swelling) and the breakdown of the blood-brain barrier (BBB) after TBI,[369] both of which can result in even more damage to the brain. I like to supplement with 600 mg of citicoline while also eating choline-rich foods like egg yolks, broccoli, and organ meats. If your healthcare provider advises higher supplementation, the Institute of Medicine (IOM) has proposed a tolerable upper intake level (maximum dose) of citicoline to be 3,500 mg/day[370] for adults (including pregnant and lactating women), but supplementation in therapeutic doses should be advised by a qualified healthcare professional.

Gastric Feed Information

I prefer to get my choline from food sources in conjunction with supplementation. While supplying choline-rich foods, we can also add powder or capsules of citicoline to gastric feeds before blending. If your healthcare provider advises higher supplementation, the upper limit (maximum dose) of citicoline is 3,500 mg/day. Supplementation in therapeutic doses should be advised by a qualified healthcare professional.

DOCOSAHEXAENOIC ACID (DHA)

Again, DHA is a kind of Omega-3 fatty acid that is largely found in fatty fish like mackerel, sardines, salmon, and tuna. As shown in the "Vegans and Vegetarians" section of the book, there are studies showing the uses of Omega-3s in waking comatose patients and accelerating neurological recovery.[371] Because they seem to have an extremely potent effect on protecting the brain, not only are sports leagues very interested in Omega-3s and their effects in preventing and treating brain injury, but scientists in the military are also inspecting this nutrient for brain injury treatment and neuroprotection. In 2011, an article in *Military Medicine*, the official journal of The Association of Military Surgeons of the United States (AMUS), wrote that "…a comprehensive, coordinated research program to evaluate the multiple uses of n-3 FA [Omega-3 fatty acids] should be a high priority for the Department of Defense."[372]

Some clinicians are hesitant to use high-dose omega-3s because there is evidence that they thin the blood. An article published in the *Journal of Neurotrama*, however, analyzes the literature and states that "[t]he overall clinical data suggests that DHA at doses up to 6 g/day does not have deleterious effects on platelet aggregation or other clotting parameters in normal individuals, and fish oil does not augment aspirin-induced inhibition of blood clotting."[373] Check with your doctor if you need to be concerned. See feedabrain.com/omega for more information.

Supplementation Information

While in the short-term, it seems like therapeutic (very high) doses of Omega-3s can be beneficial, I do not think that more than five grams per day of Omega-3s should be an ongoing practice. Additionally, the quality of the fish oil is paramount and we need to be sure that the oil is not spoiled or oxidized. For this reason, in addition to eating plenty of cold water fatty fish, I like to supplement with up to 3 grams per day of a high quality fish oil. You can find these high quality fish oils at feedabrain.com/omega, and a vegetarian source that still contains EPA and DHA can be found at feedabrain.com/vegan. You may want to check with your qualified healthcare practitioner for amounts specific to you or your loved one.

Gastric Feed Information

Supplementation in conjunction with whole food sources may be beneficial for this nutrient. When feeding through a gastric tube, in addition to including fatty fish, we can supplement using a high quality liquid fish oil like one of those found on feedabrain.com/omega. We can also use a high-powered blender like a Blendtec™ or Vitamix™ to blend a high quality fish oil supplement. Go to feedabrain.com/tools for high quality blenders. For vegans and vegetarians, we can blend an omega-3 derived from algae for a good source of EPA and DHA (feedabrain.com/vegan). Because cod liver oil is rich in many other fat-soluble vitamins such as vitamin A, cod liver oil may not be appropriate at therapeutic (very high) doses. Work with a qualified practitioner when supplementing in therapeutic doses.

URIDINE

Uridine is concentrated in broccoli, beets, mushrooms, and organ meats like liver and pancreas. It is an important nucleotide found in RNA, and while the combination of choline and DHA have shown great benefits in promoting synaptogenesis, when combined with uridine monophosphate (UMP), the most active form of uridine, those results are enhanced.[374]

In fact, uridine monophosphate has been shown in rats to enhance the neuronal outgrowth produced by brain derived neurotrophic factor (BDNF),[375] a protein that is involved in the growth of nerve cells. Thinking of our neurons as plants, John J. Ratey, MD, an associate professor of psychiatry at Harvard Medical School and author of A User's Guide to the Brain,calls the brain derived neurotrophic factor (BDNF) that is enhanced by uridine "Miracle-Gro for the brain."[376] We want our neurons to grow and thrive, so we want to supply enough uridine monophosphate.

Unfortunately, Dr. Wurtman points out that the only food that contains ingredients that can increase uridine levels in the blood is human breast milk.[377] In fact, supplemental uridine monophosphate is added to most infant formulas because of its important role in the developing brain.[378] After an injury or disease, we are rebuilding, rewiring, and re-developing our brains, so in addition to eating uridine-rich food, I like to also supplement with uridine monophosphate.[379]

Supplementation Information

While consuming uridine-rich food, such as organ meats, broccoli, beets, and nutritional yeast, if well tolerated (it's not for me), I often take 300 mg of uridine monophosphate, once or twice daily, but it is likely beneficial to ingest even more. A safety report prepared for the U.S. Food and Drug Administration in 2002 regarding the use of uridine as a supplement concluded that "[u]ridine is a rather safe drug in humans at least at doses up to 10 grams."[380]

*It is advised that you work with your qualified practitioner for specific amounts.

Gastric Feed Information

For gastric feeding, in addition to supplying uridine-rich foods, such as organ meats, broccoli, and beets, we can also add powder or capsules of uridine monophosphate to gastric feeds. According to the FDA, the upper limit is as high as 10g. Go to feedabrain.com/synapto for these supplements.

*It is advised that you work with your qualified health practitioner for specific amounts.

FEED A BRAIN SMOOTHIES

Because I feel like my brain is jump started the morning after eating or drinking a meal that contains each of the three categories of produce (leafy greens, sulfur, and brightly colored), as well as the three nutrients for synaptogenesis, I like to drink what I call a "Feed a Brain smoothie" later in the day (lunch or dinner). Because mechanisms of neuroplasticity (the brains ability to change) seem to occur at a greater extent when we are sleeping, I like to supply the building blocks for that plasticity and eat extra produce for lunch or dinner. This also helps to keep my blood sugar stable. I also like to regularly switch up the kinds of produce that I use so that my microbiome is getting a variety of different foods, which we talked about in the "Keep Switching It Up" section of the book. This handout* will help you create Feed a Brain smoothies to support brain health, while switching ingredients to keep it interesting for you, your microbiome, and your health!

* Portions of this handout are adapted from THE WAHLS PROTOCOL by Terry Wahls and Eve Adamson, copyright ©2014 by Dr. Terry Wahls L.LC. Used by permission of Avery, an imprint of Penguin Publishing Group, a division of Penguin Random House LLC.

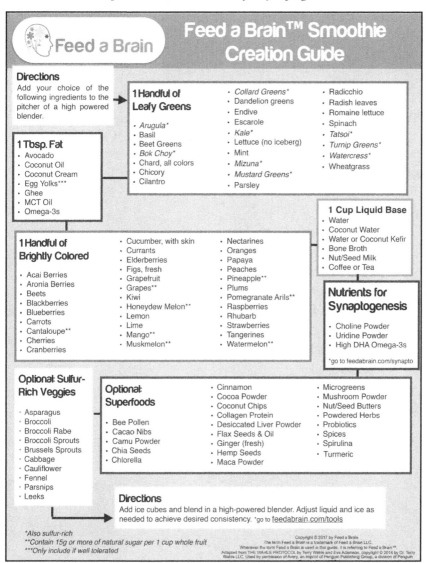

Feed a Brain™ Smoothie Creation Guide

Feed a Brain

Directions
Add your choice of the following ingredients to the pitcher of a high powered blender.

1 Tbsp. Fat
- Avocado
- Coconut Oil
- Coconut Cream
- Egg Yolks***
- Ghee
- MCT Oil
- Omega-3s

1 Handful of Leafy Greens
- *Arugula**
- Basil
- Beet Greens
- *Bok Choy**
- Chard, all colors
- Chicory
- Cilantro

- *Collard Greens**
- Dandelion greens
- Endive
- Escarole
- *Kale**
- Lettuce (no iceberg)
- Mint
- *Mizuna**
- *Mustard Greens**
- Parsley

- Radicchio
- Radish leaves
- Romaine lettuce
- Spinach
- *Tatsoi**
- *Turnip Greens**
- *Watercress**
- Wheatgrass

1 Cup Liquid Base
- Water
- Coconut Water
- Water or Coconut Kefir
- Bone Broth
- Nut/Seed Milk
- Coffee or Tea

1 Handful of Brightly Colored
- Acai Berries
- Aronia Berries
- Beets
- Blackberries
- Blueberries
- Carrots
- Cantaloupe**
- Cherries
- Cranberries

- Cucumber, with skin
- Currants
- Elderberries
- Figs, fresh
- Grapefruit
- Grapes**
- Kiwi
- Honeydew Melon**
- Lemon
- Lime
- Mango**
- Muskmelon**

- Nectarines
- Oranges
- Papaya
- Peaches
- Pineapple**
- Plums
- Pomegranate Arils**
- Raspberries
- Rhubarb
- Strawberries
- Tangerines
- Watermelon**

Nutrients for Synaptogenesis
- Choline Powder
- Uridine Powder
- High DHA Omega-3s

*go to feedabrain.com/synapto

Optional: Sulfur-Rich Veggies
- Asparagus
- Broccoli
- Broccoli Rabe
- Broccoli Sprouts
- Brussels Sprouts
- Cabbage
- Cauliflower
- Fennel
- Parsnips
- Leeks

Optional: Superfoods
- Bee Pollen
- Cacao Nibs
- Camu Powder
- Chia Seeds
- Chlorella

- Cinnamon
- Cocoa Powder
- Coconut Chips
- Collagen Protein
- Desiccated Liver Powder
- Flax Seeds & Oil
- Ginger (fresh)
- Hemp Seeds
- Maca Powder

- Microgreens
- Mushroom Powder
- Nut/Seed Butters
- Powdered Herbs
- Probiotics
- Spices
- Spirulina
- Turmeric

Directions
Add ice cubes and blend in a high-powered blender. Adjust liquid and ice as needed to achieve desired consistency. *go to feedabrain.com/tools

*Also sulfur-rich
**Contain 15g or more of natural sugar per 1 cup whole fruit
***Only include if well tolerated

Copyright © 2017 by Feed a Brain
The term Feed a Brain is a trademark of Feed a Brain LLC.
Whenever the term Feed a Brain is used in this guide, it is referring to Feed a Brain ™.
Adapted from THE WAHLS PROTOCOL by Terry Wahls and Eve Adamson, copyright © 2014 by Dr. Terry Wahls LLC. Used by permission of Avery, an imprint of Penguin Publishing Group, a division of Penguin.

HOW WILL I BE EATING?

Most of the times when I eat, I like to get all three categories of produce in roughly equal amounts. This can be done all in one meal, or with a combination of a meal (or soup) with a whole food smoothie. This is an example of a combination that supplies all of the necessary nutrients. The refreshing smoothie recipe comes from Dr. Terry Wahls' new cookbook: *Wahls Protocol Cooking for Life*, and the soup recipe is courtesy of V (paleobosslady.com).

These and other recipes can be found at feedabrain.com/recipes. Enjoy!

TERRY'S GREEN GINGER SMOOTHIE

Servings x2 (mostly greens)

Ingredients:
- 1 fist parsley (or another herb)
- 1/2 inch ginger
- 3 cups water
- 2 tbs lime juice or lemon juice
- Optional - One can coconut milk (if using coconut milk, reduce water to one cup)
- Optional - a handful of ice cubes
- 2 tbs olive oil

Combine all ingredients in a blender on high until smooth... Enjoy!

V'S CABBAGE STEW

Yield: 4 servings (mostly colored and sulfur)
Prep Time: 30 minutes
Cook Time: 45 minutes

Ingredients:
- 2 fists green cabbage: chopped
- 1 fist red cabbage: chopped
- 2 fists carrot: chopped
- 2 fists onion: chopped
- 1 fist sized sweet potato cut into rounds

MEATBALLS (optional (If not making because of egg content, use mild Italian sausage)
- 1 tbsp almond flour
- 1 pound of ground pork
- 1 large egg
- 1 large garlic clove: chopped
- 1 fist parsley: chopped
- 1 quart bone broth
- Olive oil or desired good medium or high heat fat (see Guide to Fats and Oils handout)
- Salt to taste (preferably pink Himalayan sea salt)
- Black pepper to taste

Preparation:
1. Heat a saucepan over medium heat with enough desired good fat to cover pan. Add 1 onion to oil and heat until golden in color.
2. Add cabbage, cut into big chunks to pan until golden in color (about 5 minutes). I actually like it charred a little on the edges. Once golden, then add your bone broth.

3. Cover, reduce heat to low, and simmer for about 20 minutes.
4. Slice sweet potato into rounds, and begin to make meatballs (optional - if not making, use mild Italian sausage)

MEATBALLS (skip if using sausage)

1. Add almond flour, garlic, parsley, egg, remaining onion, salt and pepper to ground pork and mix (I personally use my hands and jump right in there mixing until blended).
2. Heat cast iron or sauté pan with desired fat over medium heat.
3. Add medium size rolled meatball or whole sausage to oil. Cooking for 7 minutes turning once.
4. Remove and put aside with sweet potato rounds.
5. Check cabbage cooking until fork soft. Adding more bone broth as needed.
6. 10 minutes before serving, add meatballs or sausages cut into inch size pieces, sweet potato rounds and salt/pepper to cabbage cooking over medium with lid on pot.
7. Once potatoes are fork soft (about 5 minutes) remove from heat and serve in a large bowl.

This is a flavorful recipe full of healthy nutrients! Enjoy!

Chapter 10
THE INS — SUPERFOODS

Especially after an injury or throughout a disease process, we want to supply nutrients in ample quantities to meet the increased demands of the brain and body, and these super foods help us to do that. Some people have a hard time introducing these super foods.... I know I did. But these foods contribute significantly to our brain and body health, and they are often missing from our diets. We will consider super foods to be nutrient-rich foods that are especially beneficial for overall health as well as neurological recovery and optimization.

There are four important super foods that we will focus on here. I will also explain why these foods are important and how we can incorporate them into our diets often.

ORGAN MEATS

> **Consume about two fist-sized pieces per week. To prevent an overdose of vitamin A, consume no more than one fist-size from liver as part of your weekly animal protein allowance.**[381]

Organ meats may be the most nutrient-dense foods that we can consume, and considering the nutrients that they supply, they tend to be inexpensive. Not only do organ meats contain B vitamins, coenzyme Q10, an important factor in activating the conversion of food into energy, and all three of the important nutrients for synaptogenesis that we talked about in the last chapter (DHA, uridine, and choline), but they are also packed with important fat-soluble vitamins like A, D, E, and K.[382]

Even though they are packed with important nutrients, not all organ meats are appropriate for everyone, especially those with high iron levels. For those of us with high iron levels, we may want to limit our iron intake by avoiding foods like clams, oysters, and some organ meats like liver. We recommend that those with high iron levels work with a qualified healthcare practitioner. For healthy adults, consuming at least 12 ounces (340 grams) of organ meat a week, no more than 8 ounces (227 grams) from liver is encouraged.[383] We can simplify organ meats regarding fist size as well: about two fists of organ meat per week, no more than one fist size from liver.

If you are like I used to be, the idea of cooking and eating the liver, heart, kidneys, pancreas, etc. of an animal probably doesn't sound very appetizing. When prepared right, however, they make for a delicacy at a fancy restaurant. Unfortunately, cooking organ meats to perfection usually takes a lot of culinary skill, but we do not need to be five-star chefs to reap the benefits of these foods. You can supplement organ meats. Go to feedabrain.com/supplements for information on organ meat supplements. Go to feedabrain.com/meat for information on high quality meat, fish, organ meats, and organ meat sausages that are very nutrient rich, and palatable.

If you are still having trouble eating organ meats, these are some tricks that I've found to supply these nutrients:

Supplementation Information

Whether eating conventionally or through a gastric tube, desiccated organ meat supplements are the easiest option to supply this super food. Desiccated organ meats tend to come in capsules and are essentially ground organ meats which have had the moisture removed to preserve them. All you need to do is buy some organ meat pills and take them each day. You can find these superfood supplements at: feedabrain.com/supplements.

Gastric Feed Information

If nutrition is being provided via a gastric tube, taste is less of an issue. Liver is probably the easiest organ to purée for gastric tube feeds. Just make sure the liver is frozen for at least 14 days to kill any possible pathogens, thaw, add to any other ingredients that are to go into a tube feed (bone broth, fruits, vegetables, good fat, meat), and purée using a high-powered blender like those found at feedabrain.com/tools. Then use the Gastric Feed Creation Instructions found at feedabrain.com/handouts. Rather than pureeing the liver raw, you could also cook organ meats using the included recipes or one of the recipes on feedabrain.com/organmeat before blending, or you can simply add the powder from desiccated organ meat supplements like those found at feedabrain.com/supplements.

Freezer "Organ Meat Pills"

Save your money! You can make your own "organ meat pills" in a cheaper, safe, and even more nutritious form (with more enzymes still intact). Here's how you do it:

1. Rinse the organ meat and pat it dry before laying it on a cutting board.
2. With a sharp knife, cut the organ meat into pill-sized chunks.
3. Place the pieces, separated, on a parchment-lined cookie sheet.
4. Freeze until solid and then transfer to smaller container if desired.
5. Allow organ meat to stay frozen for 14 days before eating to kill any possible pathogens. If the organ meat was previously frozen for at least 14 days, it should be safe to eat raw or to be refrozen immediately after thawing to cut into pills. (If you're really good with a knife, you can cut frozen organ meat into pill-sized chunks without thawing, but cutting frozen meat with a knife can be very dangerous, so do not try this unless you are very confident in your knife skills).

Try to swallow a couple of these frozen organ meat "pills" every day.

Hidden Organ Meat Trick

This is also a popular trick that can be used to incorporate these superfoods:

1. Purée liver (or other organ meat) in a food processor or blender.
2. Mix the purée well with ground meat (like beef, pork, turkey, or bacon) and/or sausage.
3. Cook as desired.

For more recipes, try Googling:
"hidden (insert organ) (insert recipe type)"
For example, try Googling "hidden beef heart burgers" to find recipes, or you can find more info and organ meat recipes at feedabrain.com/organmeat.

Gastric Feed Information

If nutrition is being provided via a gastric tube, taste is less of an issue. Liver is probably the easiest organ to purée for gastric tube feeds. Make sure the liver is frozen for at least 14 days to kill any possible pathogens, thaw, add to any other ingredients that are to go into a tube feed (bone broth, fruits, vegetables, good fat, meat, etc.), and purée using a high powered blender like those found at feedabrain.com/tools. Rather than pureeing the liver raw, you could also cook organ meats using the included recipes or one of the recipes found at feedabrain.com/organmeat before blending.

FERMENTED FOODS

Include Some Amount Every Day. Fermented foods have been a part of the human diet in every habitable continent on the planet for hundreds of thousands of years.[384] A food is fermented by using a combination of yeast and bacteria in an environment that does not have oxygen (submerged in liquid). Over time, a host of bacteria are created through the fermentation process, and these bacteria protect the food from spoiling.[385] Not only that but these beneficial bacteria are also very favorable to the bacterial population of our guts, the importance of which we talked about in the "Keep Switching It Up" section.[386]

Fermented foods are the probiotics of nature. They are shown to be health-promoting by enhancing the immune system and the absorption of nutrients, decreasing the prevalence of allergies, and reducing the risk of certain cancers. Fermented foods in the diet are also a very cost-effective way for us to protect against microbial infection and disease.[387]

Some preferred (wheat and milk free) fermented foods include:
- Almond, soy (Non-GMO), and coconut yogurt
- Kombucha tea
- Beet kvass
- Water or coconut kefir
- Kimchi
- Raw sauerkraut, pickles, or other fermented vegetables

When buying fermented foods, we want to be sure that they have not been pasteurized. Pasteurization kills the beneficial bacteria, which is the main reason we want fermented foods; they are probiotic rich. Any fermented food that is not found in the refrigerated section has likely been pasteurized.[388]

Supplementation Information

Some people don't particularly like the taste of fermented foods (or currently have an undesirable reaction to them), in which case we can supplement with probiotics. While different probiotics have different effects that are useful for different conditions, as a general recommendation for wellness, I suggest soil-based organism supplements. Soil-based organism supplements are usually well tolerated. You can find more information about these supplements at feedabrain.com/superfood.

Still, some people may have a bad reaction to both fermented food *and* probiotics. If this is the case for you, remove for a few days and try to reintroduce only the tiniest bit. For fermented foods, you can try one teaspoon at a time (for probiotics, open a capsule and sprinkle a dash in your food or water). If, after at least 24 hours, you are not experiencing digestive problems, you can move on to 2 teaspoons (or 2 dashes of probiotic powder). Build up to 3 teaspoons the next day, 4 the next, and so on (or more probiotic powder). With the probiotics, try taking more of the capsule working up to the recommended dose. If you experience digestive issues, go back 1 teaspoon (or less probiotic) for a week and then try increasing, adding 1 teaspoon (or a bit more probiotic powder) to your daily intake. This will encourage a gradual shift in your bacterial makeup.

Gastric Feed Information

Because fermented foods can result in digestive issues when there is an unfavorable microbiome in the digestive system, it is important to start low and slow (1 teaspoon fermented food or one dash of probiotic powder at a time as described above) while monitoring bathroom frequency and consistency. It is advised that you work with a qualified healthcare professional.

SEA VEGETABLES

Fresh (or soaked and reconstituted): 2.5 ounces/day. One third of an ounce (or 10 g) of dried seaweed will reconstitute to about 2.5 ounces of fresh seaweed.
Dried flakes: 1 teaspoon/day
Powdered: ¼ teaspoon/day

Sea vegetables are important for many reasons, including their mineral-rich content, and one of the most important minerals found in seaweed that is hard to find elsewhere in the diet is iodine. Iodine plays an important role in many functions of the brain and body,[389] including the production and use of thyroid hormones, which direct *all* metabolism in the body,[390] and we talked earlier about the importance of metabolism.

Iodine is also good for muscle growth and for detoxing estrogen and heavy metals like lead and mercury.[391] Iodized salts have been the primary source of iodine for the US,[392] but for numerous reasons, I agree with Dr. Wahls that we should get our iodine from whole foods like sea vegetables.[393] In addition to iodine, sea vegetables contain a wealth of over a dozen important minerals like chromium, iron, manganese, magnesium, selenium, vanadium, and zinc.[394] You'll also get a variety of vitamins in the vitamin B group and vitamins A, C, E, and K. And if that wasn't enough, sea veggies help to protect us from absorbing toxic solvents, plastics, heavy metals, and even radioactivity.[395]

Just as there were different colored categories of vegetables and fruits, there are different colors in the sea veggie family. These categories are red, brown, green, and algae.[396] While it is beneficial to get any seaweed in our diets, each of these different color categories provide different benefits, so it is best to try to eat seaweeds from all of the different groups. See the sea veggie chart below or at feedabrain.com/sea.

Sea vegetables can be found at many supermarkets (just ask), and you can also order them online. Information about high-quality sea vegetables is found at feedabrain.com/sea.

The best way we can get nutrients from sea vegetables is to simply add them to our food because our taste for the food will guide how much we want to eat. We want to start slow, with a small amount, and then gradually increase the amount of sea vegetables that we consume. If you're eating your sea veggies in the form of flakes, work up to 1 teaspoon/day, for powder, ¼ teaspoon/day should be sufficient; for supplements, work up to the recommended dose; and if you have fresh seaweed, you want about 2.5 ounces (71 gram) each day.

Note: If you are taking thyroid medication, please speak with your doctor about sea veggies. The increase in iodine can necessitate a change in medicine.[397]

Supplementation Information

Go to feedabrain.com/sea for links to some supplements and flakes for each different color of sea vegetables. It is especially beneficial to get a variety of different colors of sea vegetables. The simplest is to alternate between kelp supplements and dulse supplements. Alternate with one capsule of either the kelp or the dulse every other day for a month. So, if you had a capsule of kelp on Monday, on Wednesday you would have one capsule of dulse, and back to a capsule of kelp on Friday. If by the next month you are feeling good, you can then start to alternate one capsule each day. So if you have kelp on Monday, you would have dulse on Tuesday, and then kelp again on Wednesday.

Gastric Feed Information

Powdered sea vegetables can be added to gastric feeds and alternated each day or week as needed, but because iodine is a mineral that may drastically affect thyroid function, it is important to work with a health care provider and to start low and slow. For example, you might start with ¼ teaspoon of one color of sea vegetable and alternate with a different color as often as is feasible.

SEA VEGETABLE CHART

Algae	Blue green algae Chlorella Spirulina Seaweed
Red	Dulse Flakes Irish Moss Nori
Brown	Bladderwrack Kelp Kombu Flakes Wakame
Green	Sea Lettuce

You can find information on many of these products at feedabrain.com/sea.

COLD WATER FATTY FISH

Include at least two fists per week as part of your total animal protein allowance.[398]

In recent years, many have become scared to eat fish. Contaminated waters have led to concerns about the environmental pollutants found in fish. These pollutants, like PCBs, dioxins, and mercury (to name a few) have actually been shown to cause neurological problems![399] So why is it that I advocate eating cold water fish? Because their benefits far outweigh the risks.

In 2006, a paper titled, "Fish Intake, Contaminants and Human Health: Evaluating the Risks and Benefits" was published in *JAMA: The Journal of the American Medical Association*.[400] This paper analyzed several studies examining the impact of fish consumption and it concluded: "For major health outcomes among adults...the benefits of fish intake exceed the potential risks."[401] The article goes on to demonstrate that concerns about toxins in fish have been overblown and that there is almost no risk associated with eating fish when a few simple precautions are taken.[402] As it turns out, fish do not contain very many

PCBs and dioxins when compared to meat, dairy, or vegetables.[403] The biggest takeaway message that I got from this article was that selenium, a mineral that's very rich in many fish, actually binds to mercury molecules, neutralizing them as a toxin.[404] This means that fish with more selenium than mercury do not contain the unbound form of mercury that may have adverse health effects. [405]

Most fish have plenty of selenium, especially smaller fish, and

as long as a fish has less mercury than selenium, the mercury content of the fish is not a reason to limit consumption.[406]

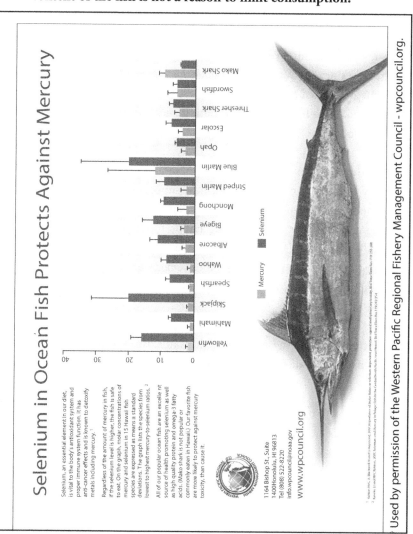

*The chart above can be found as a printable, full-size PDF file at feedabrain. com/handouts.

Smaller fish are especially safe because they tend to have less mercury and more selenium.[407] All of that being said, we want to be careful of some fish that have more mercury than selenium. These fish include some large predatory fish like pilot whale, tarpon, marlin, swordfish, and sharks.[408]

A nice fillet of wild caught Alaskan salmon, a rainbow trout, or other small fatty cold-water fish, is packed with nutrients that support the brain. There are sources of high-quality and sustainable seafood harvested from healthy, well-managed wild fisheries, offered in both frozen and even canned options. Excellent seafood can be stored in a can for a reasonable price, and as long as the fish does not get too hot, the beneficial Omega-3s stay intact. But these high-quality canned products are rarely available in local grocery stores. Go to feedabrain.com/fish for more information and a possible option for sourcing your seafood.

One of the main nutrients that fatty fish supplies is the Omega-3 fatty acid DHA. We have already talked about how supportive this nutrient is to brain health and recovery, and that sports teams and the military are even beginning to recognize its importance in treating and protecting the brains of their players and soldiers. Because Omega-3s from fish have been shown to be neuroprotective, consult this graph which shows the average Omega-3 content of common fish, so that you can favor fish with a higher Omera-3 content when choosing what to eat.

In addition to supplying plenty of cold water fish, I also like to supplement DHA through fish oils like those found at feedabrain.com/omega.

*The chart below can be found as a printable, full-size PDF file at feedabrain. com/handouts.

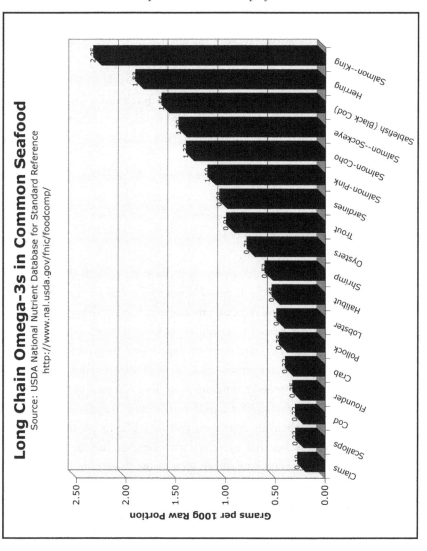

Long Chain Omega-3s in Common Seafood

Source: USDA National Nutrient Database for Standard Reference
http://www.nal.usda.gov/fnic/foodcomp/

ADDITIONAL GUIDELINES FOR BRAIN HEALTH

What we have covered so far will likely make a huge difference for most people, but for an even better prescription that further reduces the possibility of sensitivity reactions to foods that may negatively impact the brain, consider some of these guidelines as well.

- Remove or reduce grains (including non-gluten grains)
- Grains have a very high carbohydrate load without providing many brain supportive micronutrients.

- Remove or reduce mushrooms
- Mushrooms are not always well tolerated.
- Remove or reduce legumes (beans) and peanuts (peanuts are legumes)
  ◊ Not only do legumes contribute significantly to your carbohydrate intake without supplying very much brain building nutrition, but they also contain phytates (which are otherwise known as "antinutrients") compounds that hinder the absorption of certain nutrients.
- Remove or reduce all higher carbohydrate colored fruits and vegetables (see the Color Chart)
- Reduce or remove fruits and vegetables that are not on the Color Chart (like apples, bananas, and pears).
- Remove eggs
  ◊ Eggs can be beneficial, especially because of the choline in the yolks, but they can also be harmful if not well tolerated. For example, I experience gas and increased mucus as a reaction to egg whites. This suggests that I have an immune response to the food, and testing confirms this. I do not, however, experience symptoms to egg yolks.
  ◊ While some practitioners disagree with this practice because the tiniest exposure to an inflammatory food will result in an immune response, if you suspect a mild intolerance to eggs but would like to include them in your diet, you may like to try the three-step elimination diet that we talked about earlier, but for each section of the egg (whites and yolks). Here's how this would be done:
  ◊ First, try removing eggs for at least 60 days, reintroducing just the yolk (two to six egg yolks in one day depending on size, age, gender, etc.) of pasture raised eggs (less of a chance of an inflammatory response). Continue eating the yolks for a few days.
  ◊ Over the next week, check in with yourself regularly to see if you notice any changes.
  ◊ If you notice a negative effect at any point during this experiment, stop immediately. If you're working with someone who is unable to communicate, simply remove eggs from their diet, but be sure to supply choline through supplementation as well as through meat (especially organ meats), fish, broccoli, and/or collard greens. If you do not notice any changes over a week with this egg yolk experiment, you may choose to include egg yolks in your diet.

◊   After this experiment, you can try introducing the entire egg if you'd like. You don't need to wait an additional 60 days because you have already removed the entire egg for 60 days and have only introduced the egg yolk. Try introducing the entire egg in a substantial amount (two to six eggs in one day depending on size, age, gender, etc.) for a few days, waiting a week, and again, checking in with yourself regularly to see if you notice any changes.

Gastric Feed Information

When choosing food for gastric feeding, it is a good idea to also follow ALL of these additional guidelines, removing the food when the guideline says "remove or reduce." While removing these foods, be sure to supply adequate nutrition by following the portions outlined in this guide. You may want to work with a functional medicine practitioner, a functional nutritionist, or other qualified healthcare provider. Go to feedabrain.com/practitioners for a list of preferred practitioners.

Chapter 11
MOTIVATION — TO SURVIVORS AND LOVED ONES

The motivation to improve our situation is within each of us. Thoughts are powerful. By continuing to think that our or our loved one's injuries, diseases, or circumstances are all simply unfortunate and forever, we are destroying our drive. It's not that our focus on the worst-case scenario creates a bad outcome, but it gets in the way of our best-case scenario. While there is no magic pill that we can take to rehabilitate the brain, our courage and drive to implement these changes can change the course of our lives.

People often ask me if I believe that there was a reason that my life took this sharp and painful turn, implying that my brain injury and the events that followed were predestined. I do not know if that is the case, but what I do know is that I will continue to put forth the effort to give this entire ordeal a purpose and to help others to do the same.

I'm not here to give you some motivational mumbo jumbo. I'm here to give you tools and to show you the simple truth. And this is the truth: **you can do this!** You have almost certainly eaten meals in the past that did not contain milk or wheat, and you can do it again. Without even knowing it, you have probably also gotten all three of these types of produce in one meal in the past. Start with one meal free of wheat and dairy, then bring in a meal that contains each kind of produce. Incorporate supplements and nutrients for synaptogenesis. Include a super-food or two. Bit by bit, you will see the effects and you will have the resources in this guide to feed your brain nutritionally.

We need to drive our own brain health and this book can be our map. It's up to us! **Hold your head high, take the wheel, and let's bring it on home.**

Chapter 12
FOOD LABELS IN THE USA

Whether organic or conventional, what is most important is that the foods described above are supplied. That being said, I would like you to know where and how to supply the best quality nutrition as well. And because many of us shop at a grocery store in the USA, we have created a handout that outlines food labels in the US. There is a lot of confusion surrounding food labels. In fact, I have talked to farmers who were selling eggs that were labeled "cage-free," but their chickens were actually pasture-raised. Their eggs were of higher quality than advertised. This shows us that even farmers are confused about food labels; so let's go through some of the more common food labels.

Are terms like organic, grass-fed, wild caught, or pasture raised just a marketing gimmick to charge more? What about free-range, cage-free, vegetarian-fed, or all natural? After extensive research and conversations with farmers, functional practitioners, and nutritionists, it has become clear that some labels mean a lot while others don't mean much. Let's break down some food labels and meanings.

*For your convenience, all charts can be found as printable, full-size, color PDF files at feedabrain.com/handouts.

Food Labels in the USA

Feed a Brain

Are terms like organic, grass-fed, wild caught, or pasture raised just a marketing gimmick to charge more? What about free-range, cage free, vegetarian-fed, or all natural? After extensive research and conversations with farmers, functional practitioners, and nutritionists, it's become clear that some labels mean a lot while others don't mean much. Let's break down some food labels and meanings.

Disregard:

⋄'All Natural':
 * This label means almost nothing. There is no specific definition of the "Natural" label
⋄ Local:
 * There is no legal standard for the "Local" label.
⋄ Farmed or Farm Fresh:
 * This label doesn't mean anything, yet it is often used to make eggs sound more appealing.
⋄ Cage-Free or Free-Range:
 * Both Cage-Free and Free-Range still include indoor confinement for birds.
⋄ Farmed Fish:
 * Fish farms are tanks or netted areas in the ocean where fish are not able to interact with their natural environment.

WHAT PEOPLE THINK — Reality
FREE-RANGE
WHAT PEOPLE THINK — Reality
CAGE FREE

Try to get:

◆ Organic or Non-GMO fruits and vegetables
◆ Grass fed beef, lamb, buffalo, and dairy products
◆ Pasture-raised pork, chickens, turkeys, and eggs
◆ Wild caught fish

Preferred: What do they mean?

USDA ORGANIC — Organic	The "organic" label means that the food is non-GMO and that it is not grown with the use of most synthetic fertilizers and pesticides. *If the food comes from a small local farm, even if it's not certified organic, it is often better than organics being shipped in from far away!
NON GMO Project VERIFIED — Non-GMO	Organic food is always non-GMO, but non-GMO food is not necessarily organic. There are two main forms of GMO crops: herbicide resistant and pesticide producing. It has been shown that GMO crops provide fewer nutrients.
CERTIFIED GRASSFED — Grass-Fed	The "Grass Fed" Label This label means that for most of the animal's life, it was free to graze for its own fresh food rather than being fed by a feedbag or trough. The idea behind grass fed animals is to allow them to eat the closest thing to their natural diet as possible. Look for packages labeled, "100% grass fed." Go to feedabrain.com/meat.
Pasture Raised — Pasture Raised	Pasture-raised poultry is a sustainable technique in which birds or other omnivores are actually able to roam on a large pasture, as opposed to indoor confinement. Both cage-free and free-range are still indoor confinement for birds. Pastured, or pasture raised is the kind of pork, eggs, chicken, turkey, and other poultry that we want.
Wild Caught	Fish farms are tanks or netted areas in the ocean where fish are not able to interact with their natural environment. Instead of the fish being free to roam and to eat their natural diets, they have been fed a diet that they did not evolve with. Wild caught fish are preferable. Go to feedabrain.com/fish.

BREAKDOWN

Try to get:

- Organic or Non-GMO fruits and vegetables
- Grass-fed beef, lamb, buffalo, and dairy products
- Pasture raised pork, chickens, turkeys, and eggs
- Wild caught fish

Disregard:
- All Natural
  - ◊ There is no legal definition of the "Natural" label.
- Local
  - ◊ There are no legal standards for the "Local" label.[409]
- Farmed or Farm Fresh
  - ◊ This label doesn't necessarily mean anything, yet it is often used to make eggs sound more appealing.
- Cage-Free or Free-Range
  - ◊ Both cage-free and free-range labels are still indoor confinement for birds.
- Farmed Fish
  - ◊ Fish farms are tanks or netted areas in the ocean where fish cannot interact with their natural environment.

ALL NATURAL
This label means almost nothing.

There is no specific definition of the "Natural" label. In general, "the FDA has considered the term "natural" to mean that nothing artificial or synthetic (including all color additives regardless of source) has been included in, or has been added to, a food that would not normally be expected to be in that food."[410] Unfortunately, the label says nothing about how the food was processed or manufactured.[411] The label must include a statement explaining the meaning of the term "natural" (such as "no artificial ingredients" or "minimally processed").[412]

A food that is genetically modified, administered antibiotics and hormones, fed an unnatural diet, and factory farmed in crowded conditions could still potentially carry the label "All Natural." [413]

LOCAL
This label does not necessarily mean anything.

There are no legal standards for the "local" label, so a grocery in Texas could potentially sell melons from Guatemala and call them "local" with no repercussions.[414] Shop at a store that has a reputation to protect, because the law is too loose to protect you.

That being said, if we are aware that the food comes from a small local farm, even if it's not certified organic, it is often better than big farm organics shipped in from far away! Organic certification is a long, tedious, and expensive process which may be cost-prohibitive for some small family farms.

FARM RAISED VS WILD CAUGHT FISH
Wild caught fish are preferable.

Fish farms are tanks or netted areas in the ocean where fish cannot interact with their natural environment. Instead of the fish being free to roam and to eat their natural diets, they have been fed a diet that they did not evolve with. Wild caught fish are preferable.

CAGE-FREE, FREE-RANGE, & PASTURE RAISED
Try to get pasture raised eggs and to not support the indoor confinement of birds labeled "cage-free" or "free-range."

These labels are found on poultry and eggs but what do they actually mean?

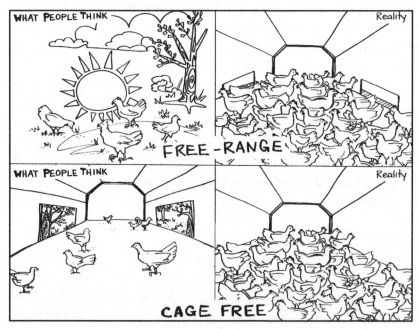

Free-range conjures up images of an open range for the birds to roam, but what free-range actually looks like is much different. The U.S. Department of Agriculture's (USDA) guidelines[415] only require producers of free-range chickens or eggs to demonstrate to the agency that the poultry has been allowed access to the outside. But, according to the Humane Society of the United States (HSUS), "no information on stocking density, the frequency or duration of how much outdoor access must be provided, nor the quality of the land accessible to the animals is defined." [416] There usually are a few doors that go to a tiny, closet-sized yard for hundreds of chickens or more that are so congested that many may never see the light of day.[417]

Cage-free is even less desirable. It is the same as free-range, except that the birds are not even given access to a small outdoor area.

Pastured, or pasture raised (not to be confused with "pasteurized"), poultry is a sustainable agriculture technique in which birds or other omnivores are actually able to roam on a large pasture, as opposed to indoor confinement.

- **Both cage-free and free-range are still indoor confinement for birds.**
- **Pastured, or pasture raised is the kind of pork, eggs, chicken, turkey, and other poultry that we want.**

NON-GMO

This label tells us that the produce is not genetically modified. But why does it matter?

There are two main forms of GMO crops: herbicide resistant and pesticide producing. Farmers want to get rid of any weeds among their crops, so herbicide resistant fruits and vegetables are planted. These plants are genetically modified to be able to survive when sprayed heavily with an herbicide called Roundup (or glyphosate), while the unmodified weeds around these plants are killed by the toxic herbicide.[418] Though it sounds like you can simply wash the glyphosate off of the produce, studies imply that the herbicide soaks into the plant, and no matter how much we scrub the produce, the toxic herbicide cannot be washed off.[419] Also, it has been shown that plants bred to be resistant to Roundup are inefficient at absorbing minerals from the soil, so we get fewer nutrients from herbicide resistant GMO crops.[420]

The other kind of genetically modified crop is called pesticide producing. This is a genetic modification in which the food itself produces toxins that kill insects when ingested.[421] It does so by damaging their digestive tracks, which contributes to intestinal permeability in rats[422] and is also likely a cause of leaky gut in humans.[423]

In April 2015, *Time Magazine* published several charts in an article called "These Charts Show Every Genetically Modified Food People Already Eat in the U.S."[424] While this article does not speak into the harms of GMOs, it is helpful to know which US crops are commonly genetically modified. You can find these charts at feedabrain.com/gmo. Over 90% of all soybean, cotton, and corn acreage in the U.S. is used to grow genetically engineered crops,[425] but other food crops that are approved to be genetically modified include sugar beets, alfalfa, canola, papaya, and other crops listed below (in order of most common to least common).

1- Corn	6- Summer Squash
2- Soybean	7- Canola
3- Cotton	8- Alfalfa
4- Potato	9- Apple
5- Papaya	10- Sugarbeet

Organic food is always Non-GMO, but Non-GMO food is not necessarily organic.

ORGANIC
Organic fruits, vegetables, and grains.
The "organic" label, when found on fruits, vegetables, and grains means that the food is Non-GMO and that it is not grown with the use of most synthetic fertilizers and pesticides. For a farm to become USDA certified organic, however, it is a long, tedious, and expensive process which may be cost prohibitive for some small family farms. Because of this, it may be better to get local food that we *know* to be from a small local farm that does not use GMO seeds.

Additionally, there are some excellent companies that provide quality products that are not yet certified. Vital Farms, for example, a collective of farms that meet a rigorous set of standards to guarantee that all of their eggs are pasture raised, buys eggs not only from certified organic farms, but also from farms that are not yet certified by the USDA. Vital Farms inspects these farms to be sure that they are up to *their* standards, which in some ways, are stricter than the USDA's standards. These eggs, which are sold as Non-GMO, are reduced a bit in price, which means that we can get quality eggs at a good price.

Organic Meat

The "organic" label, when found on meat products, means that the animal was raised on organic feed, without the use of antibiotics, which is great, but that feed still may have been an unhealthy diet. For example, "organic beef" may be fed organic grain, which is not what cattle has evolved eating. Another example is that "organic chicken" or any other poultry may be raised in congested confinement while being fed organic feed. This is why, when it comes to meat, we can do better than organic. We want:

- Grass-fed beef, lamb, buffalo, and dairy products
- Pasture raised pork, chickens, turkeys, and eggs
- Wild caught fish

VEGETARIAN-FED

Vegetarian-Fed pork, chickens, turkey, or eggs are not desirable.

The "Vegetarian-Fed" label is often coupled with an "organic" label. I usually see this on poultry, and I tend to disregard it because chickens, turkeys, and cornish game hens are not vegetarians, but omnivores that are free to eat bugs. I have noticed that sometimes farmers are confused about food labels, so when I see this label at a farmers market, I double check to see if the chickens, turkeys, pork, etc. are actually pasture raised. We do not want an animal raised on diet that it did not evolve eating, so we do not want vegetarian-fed omnivores. A vegetarian-fed pig, chicken, or turkey is a vegetarian-fed omnivore.

GRASS-FED

Grass-fed beef, buffalo, sheep, or goat is desirable.

The "Grass-Fed" Label is usually found on beef, buffalo, sheep, and goats. This label tells us that for *most* of the animal's life, it was free to graze for its own fresh food rather than being fed by a feedbag or trough. The idea behind grass-fed animals is to allow them to eat the closest thing to their natural diet as possible. But the "Grass-Fed" label is still not the best we can get. The label means that for *most* of the animal's life it was allowed to graze for its own fresh food, but most cattle are sent to a separate facility to be slaughtered, and at this facility, the cows are usually fed corn or grains that are not part of their natural diet. While we may think that this relatively short period of time would not make a difference, as it turns out, the nutrient profile, particularly the fatty acid profile, of the meat is changed for the worse.[426]

The best you can get is not only grass-fed, but also grass-finished. If the packaging says 100% grass-fed, it is also grass-finished. Ideally, this is how we want to get our cattle, buffalo, sheep, and goats: 100% grass-fed.

Chapter 13
GASTRIC FEEDING GUIDELINES AND TIPS

When we eat, the first phase of digestion occurs in the mouth where we chew our food and mix it with saliva. This chewed food then needs to be swallowed into the stomach, and not inhaled into the lungs. After a brain injury or other neurological condition, swallowing often becomes a problem, which can pose a very dangerous situation. If the pharynx, or swallowing mechanism, is not working effectively, food may enter the lungs, which could lead to life threatening infections like pneumonia. A gastric feed (also known as tube feed) is a liquid diet that is fed through a tube which bypasses the pharynx and allows for liquid nutrition to be fed into the esophagus or directly into the stomach. This is where the next phase of digestion begins. This tube is known as a gastric tube.

MY GASTRIC FEED EXPERIENCE
After I awoke from a coma, my swallowing mechanism was not working effectively, and I had contracted both pneumonia and a MRSA infection as a result. I was only permitted to eat a puréed diet by mouth. At this time, the first real food that I could enjoy orally was soup that my mom would pick up from a cafe and purée in a blender.

Unfortunately, my swallowing difficulties got worse, and I continued to aspirate my food. To bypass the possibility of me aspirating and potentially contracting another life threatening infection, a gastric tube was placed. This is a very common procedure after a TBI. I was then being fed through a gastric tube, where I received the hospital processed liquid formula that is typically fed to patients. Surprisingly, these processed liquid formulas contain many ingredients that have been shown to contribute to inflammation and/or neurodegeneration (ingredients like corn syrup,[427] canola oil,[428] soy protein isolate,[429] etc.)! Check the ingredients list of what is being fed to you or your loved one. I think you may be surprised, just as I was.

These ingredients are similar to those found in a candy bar, but this is not like having one candy bar every now and then... this is breakfast, lunch, and dinner for months, or even years for some patients! This kind of processed liquid formula is typically fed to patients who are not eating conventionally both in the hospital setting and in hospice. So, in effect, some people are essentially fed fortified corn syrup every day as their primary source of nutrition. I was one of those people.

I believe these formulas disregard the patient's overall health and well-being. In my opinion, it is almost criminal that they are routinely fed to patients. This is why a major objective of the book is to influence a positive change in hospital nutrition, especially in gastric feeds. I believe that through patient education, empowerment, and demand, we can create that change.

Nutrition is where we derive many of the building blocks needed to rebuild and repair the brain and body, so we want to supply the best nutrition that we can, especially after an injury or throughout a disease process.

TUBE FEEDING OMEGA-3s

Our primary goal is to change the feed to something of much higher quality (which we will outline in the following pages), but in conjunction with that (and possibly more importantly), there is another step that can be taken to improve brain health immensely. Research shows us numerous cases that establish high-quality Omega-3s as being especially therapeutic after a brain injury. As we talk about in the "DHA Use in Treating TBI" section of this book, high-dose fish oils, especially those high in both EPA and DHA, have been shown to powerfully support TBI recovery and neuroprotection.[430]

High-quality Omega-3s may be the most important supplementation we can take after a brain injury, especially if you or your loved one is receiving a conventional gastric feed formula. Many people have been successful in requesting that doctors allow supplementation of high-quality fish oils in the gastric tube, even if efforts to allow a blenderized tube feed (as described below) were not approved by the hospital or doctors. If real-food gastric feeds are not approved, fish oil supplementation alone can make a huge difference in recovery from a brain injury or other neurological condition. You can use the letter to clinicians further below to make the request to your doctor to allow such supplementation. You have a right to have such requests respected by the healthcare team, but remember to always strive to work collaboratively.

My passion for helping to get your loved one high-quality nutrition while in or out of the hospital is immense, so please don't hesitate to reach out for support. I offer one-on-one consultations at feedabrain.com/consult, and we are creating courses and other resources at feedabrain.com/education.

BLENDERIZED TUBE FEEDS

When I was finally discharged from the hospital, I was still receiving nutrition through a gastric tube, but I no longer had to ingest that horrible processed stuff. My mother began to make puréed soups again to put through my gastric tube by using a large syringe and a blender. This is known as a blenderized tube feed -- a real food purée administered through a gastric tube. I saw a difference in my energy levels and in my overall recovery once I was being fed a real food diet instead of the processed liquid formula.

In writing this section of the book, I consulted with Laura Schoenfeld, MPH, RD, a Registered Dietitian with a Masters in Public Health Nutrition (MPH) who has a strong background in functional medicine. For Laura's Master's thesis, in 2013 she published a paper entitled "The Use of Blenderized Tube Feeding in Pediatric Patients: Evidence and Guidelines for Dietetic Practice."[431] I also consulted with Kathryn Hayes CCC-SLP, Katy Haldiman RN (The Paleo Nurse), and Jeremy Lampel, MS, RD, CDE, a registered dietitian and certified diabetes educator with a Master's degree in nutritional science. In December of 2014, *Practical Gastroenterology* published an article titled "Blenderized Tube Feeding: Suggested Guidelines to Clinicians."[432] The PDF of this and Laura's Master's thesis can be found at feedabrain.com/gastric, and you can print them out to share with your medical team.

The Blenderized Tube Feeding: Suggested Guidelines to Clinicians article mentioned above states:

"...the best candidate is a patient and/or caregiver who made the decision to 'try' this feeding option, and is willing to commit their time and effort for instruction and preparation of BTF [Blenderized Tube Feed]."[433]

The article above explains how a supporter who is willing to commit the time can work with those who are on the patient's healthcare team (i.e. nurses, dietitians, and SLPs) to feed a patient in this manner.[434] Soon after an injury is a vulnerable period in which nutrition is vitally important. This importance is unfortunately often overlooked.[435]

In the handout on the next page, I have adapted the information in these articles to the Feed a Brain guidelines. After determining whether blenderized tube feeding is appropriate, you can use this handout to deliver foods to this guide's specifications for patients who are unable to eat conventionally. You can also purchase Feed a Brain-approved feeds and meal replacement shakes that can be fed through a gastric tube. These feeds are not as beneficial as the blenderized tube feeds outlined, but they are certainly easier to implement and are still much more beneficial than the standard hospital feed. Visit feedabrain. com/feeds to see what meal replacement and gastric feed options are available. If you are looking for optimal nutrition and have the time and energy to make your own blenderized feed, follow the instructions outlined in the Gastric Tube Feed Creation Instructions Handout* on the next page For your convenience, full-sized copies of all handouts can be found at feedabrain.com/handouts.

*Portions of this handout are adapted from THE WAHLS PROTOCOL by Terry Wahls and Eve Adamson, copyright ©2014 by Dr. Terry Wahls L.LC. Used by permission of Avery, an imprint of Penguin Publishing Group, a division of Penguin Random House LLC.

 # Gastric Tube Feed Creation Instructions
Feed a Brain

You can purchase Feed a Brain approved gastric feeds at feedabrain.com/feeds

- Ingredients

In the pitcher of a blender, or in a container that can be used with a stick blender*, add the following ingredients (to avoid food intolerances, including those caused by leaky gut, do not use any products that contain grains (including corn), dairy, egg, beans, or any artificial flavors, colors, or preservatives, and steer clear of nightshades and mushrooms.

- Carbohydrates: Three Kinds of Produce

Add equal amounts of each kind of produce (leafy greens, colors, sulfur) to the pitcher of a blender.

Roughly 2-3 fist-sized portion of each kind of produce per day

*A more extensive list of ingredients can be found in the "Guide to Greens and Sulfur-Rich Vegetables" chart. (FeedaBrain.com/handouts)

About 0.1 - 0.15oz/lbs (6-9g/kg) of body weight per day.
This is roughly equal to 2-3 portions of about the size of the individual's hand formed into a closed fist.

Leafy Greens	**Sulfur Veggies**	**Colored**	
Lettuce (no iceberg)	Broccoli	*Oranges	Melons
Spinach	Brussels sprouts	*Grapefruits	Celery
Arugula	Garlic	Beets	Carrots
Kale	Onions, all colors	Berries	Asparagus
Mustard Greens	Radishes	Grapes	Avocado
etc ...	Turnips	*Squash	Zucchini (with skin)

- Protein

Add any cooked meat or fish that is well tolerated by the patient. General macronutrient guidelines tend to be measured as grams of the macronutrient protein, but not grams of a protein containing food (like meat). Some dietician like to use this guideline as a ballpark:

Roughly 1-3 fist-sized pieces of meat per day

0.06 - 0.09 ounces of meat per pound of body weight (3.69 grams - 5.67 grams of meat per kg of body weight) per per day.
Red meat, especially organ meat, and fatty fish like salmon is desirable

If vegetarian or vegan, use foods with complete amino acid profiles (avoid soy) and work with a dietitian. Keep in mind that vegetarian sources of protein are not optimal because they also contain carbohydrates, which may replace the carbohydrates from the amount of brain-building produce that we want to consume

- Fat

Fat is very important to brain health and recovery. Supply essential Omega-3 and Omega-6 fatty acids (favor Omega-3s) using the "Brain-Supportive Fats and Oils" on the chart below:

Only use fats on this list. Do not use canola oil, vegetable oil, corn oil, cottonseed oil, grape-seed oil, peanut oil, "buttery spreads", hydrogenated or partially hydrogenated oils, trans fats, margarine, vegetable shortening, rapeseed oil, rice bran oil, safflower oil, soybean oil, sunflower oil, or wheat germ oil. Do not heat oils above smoke temp specified below.

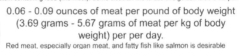

Avocado Oil (520° F)	Macadamia Oil (390° F)	Fish Oil (not for cooking)
Ghee (482° F)	Poultry & Duck Fat (375° F)	Cod Liver Oil (not for cooking)
Palm Oil (450° F)	Extra Virgin Olive Oil (375° F)	Flaxseed Oil (not for cooking)
Almond Oil (430° F)	Coconut Oil (350° F)	MCT Oil (not for cooking)
Tallow (420° F)	Sesame Oil (350° F)	Truffle Oil (not for cooking)
Lard (390° F)	Cocoa Butter (not for cooking)	

We can get our Omega-3s from liquid fish oils, or we can use capsules in a high power blender. Because Omega-3s have been shown to be neuroprotective in high dosages. You can find these supplements at feedabrain.com/omega)

*For a vegetarian option that still supplies adequate EPA and DHA, go to feedabrain.com/algae

- Directions

Add produce, fat, and protein to a container and fill with water or bone broth until most of the solid food is submerged. Use either stick blender* or a heavy duty blender found (like those found on feedabrain.com/blenders) to purée the ingredients, adding more water or bone broth if needed to get the feed to the right consistency. Let the feed come to a comfortable temperature and use a large syringe to push the formula through the gastric tube as a bolus.

*A stick blender or regular blender may be used, but the feed must be strained through a wire mesh strainer before serving (which removes some fiber)

IS A BLENDERIZED GASTRIC DIET APPROPRIATE?

How do you determine if you or your loved one is a candidate for a blenderized gastric diet? The first thing that must be considered is whether the patient is medically approved to receive bolus feeds.

In order for the feeds suggested in this guide to be used the patient must be approved for bolus gastric feeds, or feeds in which the amount of food that would be consumed in a meal is fed through a gastric tube over the course of a few minutes as opposed to a continuous feed where a small amount is trickled into the patient's stomach over hours. Bolus feeding is only appropriate with a gastrostomy (G-tube), such as a PEG tube or NG tube (both of these tubes feed into the stomach), and is not appropriate for a jejunostomy, or J tube (tube that feeds into the small intestine).

If bolus feeding is approved then we can move on to the other important considerations:
- Is someone available to support and guide this kind of feeding?
- Is someone motivated and willing to commit the time to prepare the foods or to order powdered or real food meal replacement drinks. These meals can be found at feedabrain.com/feeds.
- Are refrigeration, the use of a heavy duty blender, airtight storage containers, and ingredients (if applicable) accessible to you? Many of these items can be found at feedabrain.com/tools.

Making the Request

After thinking of all of the above considerations, patients and loved ones should seek medical permission. In a hospital setting, you will need the approval of the hospital and cooperation of the staff to implement these practices. While this may be frustrating, hospital resistance to this kind of feeding may be overcome by creating a partnership with the healthcare team. Approach your loved one's healthcare team with compassion and a desire to partner for the patient's well-being.

Personalize the patient and become aligned with the healthcare team. Find out who the dietitian is and try to make friends. If you don't have access to the dietitian, find someone on your loved one's healthcare team who seems to be compassionate and express to them why your loved one matters to you. Once you have created more interest in the person who is receiving the gastric feed, you can tell the healthcare professional what you have learned from this book and what concerns you have. After all, at the end of the day, you all share the same goal: for the patient to get better.

You can tell the dietitian or other healthcare provider what you would like to do for your loved one and why. As the conversation proceeds, you will be ready to present this clinician letter (feedabrain.com/clinicianletter) and the Feed a Brain approved gastric feeds (feedabrain.com/feeds). If more resources are needed, you can also provide the Gastric Tube Feed Creation Instructions, the two above articles concerning blenderized tube feeds (feedabrain.com/gastric), and/or the research regarding Omega-3s (feedabrain.com/omega).

Show that you are willing to put in the effort and ask if implementation of these guidelines is a realistic option. Don't expect an immediate answer, but ask them to look it over so you may discuss it the next day. You may be too busy to prepare these meals every day, which is why we are providing the option for Feed a Brain approved meal replacements to be used in a gastric feed. Some of these other options, which we believe are far superior to the conventional formulas that are usually administered, can be found at feedabrain.com/feeds. Remember that food is either helpful or harmful to us. The guidelines outlined illustrate exactly how we can feed the cells in our brains and bodies, and how we can take care of our cells so that they can take care of us.

I wrote the next two sections for clinicians on your loved ones' healthcare team who have shown compassion for your request. You can get the printable version of the letter to clinicians with citations at feedabrain.com/clinicianletter.

GASTRIC FEED CONSIDERATIONS FOR CLINICIANS

The chart below is adapted from the article written by Laura Schoenfeld, MPH, RD concerning blenderized tube feeding in pediatric patients. It details step-by-step considerations for determining if blenderized tube feeding is appropriate for a patient. In it, if we change the word "parent" to "patient or caregiver," the same criteria applies to patients of any age. This is a list of the minimum criteria for clinicians to consider before switching to a blenderized tube feed for a patient.

115

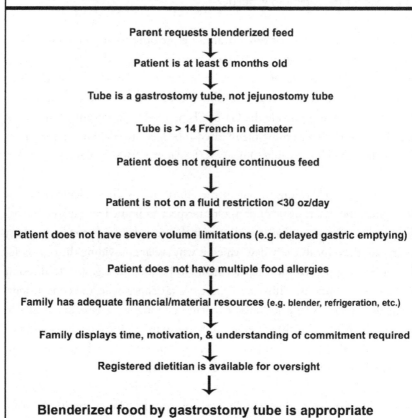

Considerations for Determining if Blenderized Tube Feeding is Appropriate

Parent requests blenderized feed
↓
Patient is at least 6 months old
↓
Tube is a gastrostomy tube, not jejunostomy tube
↓
Tube is > 14 French in diameter
↓
Patient does not require continuous feed
↓
Patient is not on a fluid restriction <30 oz/day
↓
Patient does not have severe volume limitations (e.g. delayed gastric emptying)
↓
Patient does not have multiple food allergies
↓
Family has adequate financial/material resources (e.g. blender, refrigeration, etc.)
↓
Family displays time, motivation, & understanding of commitment required
↓
Registered dietitian is available for oversight
↓
Blenderized food by gastrostomy tube is appropriate

If the patient is a realistic candidate for these gastric feeds, to better support brain function and repair, we can order Feed a Brain approved gastric feeds (feedabrain.com/feeds). If making our own blenderized feeds, follow the instructions outlined in the Gastric Tube Feed Creation Instructions Handout on page 113 and also available online. For your convenience, printable PDF copies of all handouts and charts can be found at feedabrain.com/handouts.

A LETTER TO CLINICIANS

To clinicians,

I first want to acknowledge and thank you for being open to helping families provide their loved ones with a better chance at recovery through nutrition. As you know, food is where we derive the building blocks for the function and repair of our brain and body. Powerful changes can be made for your patient's health through nutrition and supplementation.

My name is Cavin and my intention is to improve gastric feed nutrition for patients. In 2011, I sustained a TBI -- a severe Diffuse Axonal Injury. Statistically, over 90% of patients with this injury never regain consciousness. For months after waking from a coma, I didn't eat, walk, or talk, my left hand was completely flexed inward, I was breathing through a tracheotomy, and I was receiving nutrients through a PEG tube in my belly. At one point in my recovery, I was steered towards a nutritional protocol and I began to regain mental clarity. For over six years since then, I have been studying neuro-metabolism, nutrients involved in neuroplasticity, and other aspects that influence brain function. I have collaborated with practitioners of many different specialties in order to better understand our brain function, and what safe and effective interventions can be utilized to optimize patient outcomes. My recovery has been called miraculous and I owe that in large part to nutrition. Now I help others with brain injury and neurodegenerative disease. You can learn more about me at FeedaBrain.com and AdventuresinBrainInjury.com.

As a clinician, you may hold the keys to unlock a patient's recovery by advocating for better nutrition. Recovery can be supported through (1) fish oil supplementation and (2) real food blenderized gastric tube feeds.

Fish Oil Supplementation

Possibly the most powerful therapy that we can do for a brain-injured patient is to introduce high dose fish oils into their diet, especially those high in both EPA and DHA. Research shows the importance of this nutrient to brain health, brain injury treatment, and neuroprotection. In 2011, an article in Military Medicine, the official journal of The Association of Military Surgeons of the United States (AMUS), wrote that "…a comprehensive, coordinated research program to evaluate the multiple uses of n-3 FA [Omega-3 fatty acids] should be a high priority for the Department of Defense." (Lewis, Michael D. and Julian Bailes. "Neuroprotection for the warrior: dietary supplementation with omega-3 fatty acids," *Military Medicine* 176.10 (2011): 1120-127). Additionally, in 2013, the American Journal of Emergency Medicine presented a case study about a teenager who suffered a severe TBI and was given an initial GCS of 3. Ten days after the injury, he was given a large dose (15 ml, which is about 13 g) twice a day (30 mL/day) of a high-quality fish oil via his PEG. On the 21st day, he was weaned off of the ventilator, and soon progressed from vegetative state to attending his high school graduation three months later. (Lewis, Michael, et al. "Therapeutic use of omega-3 fatty acids in severe head trauma," *The American Journal of Emergency Medicine* 31.1 (2013): 273. e5-273. e8). This is not an isolated case, as other TBI survivors have also obtained similar results which you can read more about at feedabrain.com/omega.

What About the Risk of Blood Thinning?

Some clinicians are hesitant to use high-dose fish oils because there is evidence that they may thin the blood. An article published in the *Journal of Neurotrauma*, however, analyzes the literature and states that "[t]he overall clinical data suggests that DHA at doses up to 6 g/day does not have deleterious effects on platelet aggregation or other clotting parameters in normal individuals, and fish oil does not augment aspirin-induced inhibition of blood clotting." (Hasadsri, L., et al. "Omega-3 Fatty Acids as a Putative Treatment for Traumatic Brain Injury," *Journal of Neurotrauma* 30(11) (2013): 897-906. doi:10.1089/neu.2012.2672). Therefore, fish oil supplementation in doses up to 6 g/day does not appear to have the blood thinning effects that had raised concerns.

We have organized much research on the subject of Omega-3s and their effects in preventing and treating brain injury at feedabrain.com/omega.

Real Food Blenderized Tube Feeds

Surprisingly, most enteral formulas fed today contain processed ingredients like corn syrup, canola oil, sugar, corn maltodextrin, and soy protein isolate. Many of these ingredients have been shown to contribute to neurodegeneration and inflammation. These ingredients are not quality nutrition for anyone to live on, let alone someone who needs to heal after injury or throughout a disease process. Instead of using these feeds, we can use tube feeds based on real food nutrition to better support your patient's recovery and health.

There is a convenient handout showing the "Considerations for Determining if Blenderized Tube Feeding is Appropriate" available online for your use at feedabrain.com/gastric. When it comes to creating or purchasing real food gastric feeds, we have created a "Gastric Tube Feed Creation Instructions" handout, which can also be found at feedabrain.com/gastric. In addition, we have gathered a list of available premade feeds at feedabrain.com/feeds. We believe these types of feeds provide superior nutrients for brain health and recovery when compared to processed formulas.

Collaboration for the Patient's Well-Being

Both you, and the loved ones of the person you are caring for, want the patient to get better, so I hope that you are open to allowing (or requesting) that your patients be administered fish oils and/or to be fed the real food feeds outlined here.

Additionally, we are building a team of collaborative medical professionals to influence change. Together, we can make a positive change in the standard model of neurorehabilitation, and we can help to prevent neurological degeneration for everyone. If your heart breaks as you watch patients deteriorate on the currently-used feeds, I ask you to join us in this quest to improve hospital and gastric feed nutrition by signing up at feedabrain.com/collaborate.

I have so much appreciation for your profession and the work you do for patients every day. Thank you for your time and attention. I hope this information will be useful to you in the treatment of your patients.

Sincerely,

Cavin Balaster

FeedaBrain.com

AdventuresinBrainInjury.com

Author of *How to Feed a Brain: Nutrition for Optimal Brain Function and Repair*

PRACTICAL TIPS FOR GASTRIC FEEDING

Since I had a gastric tube myself, I learned a few things that make it easier. I can share a few helpful, practical tips based upon my own experience.

Blenders

In order to make these feeds to a consistency that can reliably be fed through a gastric tube, one of the tools needed is a high-powered and high-quality blender like a Blendtec™ or Vitamix™. Their abilities are quite impressive and they each come with a several-year warranty. You can find these blenders at feedabrain.com/tools.

Lower quality blenders cannot blend the food to the smooth consistency needed for tube feeding, so the tube can get clogged. In a hospital setting, the smooth consistency is imperative. It is also highly-recommended if feeding at home, since cleaning a clogged gastric tube is a time-consuming and difficult ordeal.

I never thought I would spend hundreds of dollars on a blender, but my Blendtec™ has changed my life by allowing me to get more things done with less time in the kitchen. I can swallow without any restrictions these days, so I don't need my meals blenderized, but I also enjoy these foods even as smoothies and pureed soups (usually when I'm too busy to cook). I still cook when I want to cook, go out to dinner, and regularly eat delicious meals, but I no longer have any reason to not get in the produce I know is optimal for brain function and repair.

Storage

If there is left over after first feed, seal in a container and refrigerate for use within 24 hours. If feed is not going to be used for over 24 hours, freeze for later use and then use within 12 hours of thawing.

Enzymes and Gastric Feeding

Again, gastric tubes skip the first stage of digestion when the food is chewed and mixed with saliva in the mouth. Saliva is important because it contains special enzymes, namely amylase, an enzyme that breaks down complex carbohydrates into simple sugars to prepare the food for the next phase of digestion in the stomach. Because we are skipping this step, we are going to want to add digestive enzymes to our gastric feed. For products that are designed to include important enzymes especially for when the first stage of digestion is skipped (like in gastric feeds), go to feedabrain.com/enzymes.

While enzymes can be very beneficial, Dr. Wahls and I have discussed this topic, and we both agree that nothing beats the real thing. With this in mind, let's talk about a method that can be done in addition to, or in place of, digestive enzymes.

The best way we can mimic the first stage of digestion that is bypassed in gastric feeds is to collect our saliva throughout the day and add it to our smoothies and blended soups (after they've cooled). I know it may sound gross, but by holding digestive bitters in the mouth or by chewing on something bitter (like kale or mustard greens), saliva production is encouraged, which can be added to gastric feeds for better digestion, especially if gastric feeding is long term. Either drop a few drops of digestive bitters in the mouth or chew on kale or another bitter green about 30 times. Then spit out the mixture of saliva with digestive bitters or greens to add to a soup or smoothie. Dr. Wahls says that adding 1-2 tablespoons of saliva to your tube feedings is beneficial, but any amount is helpful.

Chapter 14
A SUMMARY OF THE FEED A BRAIN MEAL PLAN

Congratulations! I am honored that you made it through this entire book! You now have so many of the nutritional tools that I use to help me to reclaim my brain by reducing brain inflammation and supplying the nutrients needed for the brain to repair and function optimally. Now it's time to put it all to use!

I can imagine that you may feel overwhelmed right now. All of the changes that you'll need to make to optimally feed your brain probably seem intimidating. I get it. This is a load of information to implement. The good news is that we don't need to implement it all at once. We can take it one step at a time. We can start by ridding our homes of the foods that we want to avoid or eliminate. That will drastically limit our exposure to the foods that do not substantially support our brain health. We can begin to supplement some of the superfoods, the nutrients for synaptogenesis, compounds to support ketogenic metabolism, and supplements to quell brain inflammation. We can start to batch cook the sulfur and colored produce and to add them to some leafy greens with meats. We can make soups, salads, and smoothies that supply much of the produce, fat, and meat that our brains need for optimal function and repair. I also offer one-on-one consultations at feedabrain.com/consult, and we are creating courses and other resources at feedabrain.com/education.

FEED A BRAIN REVIEW
To recap, let's go over some of the key points and some tools that will make this meal plan realistic and effective.

The Outs

- Remove or reduce processed foods, fast foods, and soda, even "diet" soda (sparkling water is okay).
- Remove or reduce refined sugar (like white and brown sugar).
- Remove or reduce high-fructose corn syrup.[436]
- Remove or reduce additives, artificial sweeteners, and MSG.[437, 438]
- Remove or reduce all vegetable oils like canola, soybean, corn, and grape seed.[439] (see the Guide to Fats and Oils handout)
- Remove or reduce grains (corn is a grain and is also often genetically modified). [440]
- Limit starchy vegetables and high glycemic fruits.
- Remove or reduce squeezed juice (not a whole food because the fibrous pulp has been discarded).
- Avoid all artificial trans fat, including hydrogenated or partially hydrogenated oil.[441]
- Remove milk[442, 443] and wheat[444, 445, 446, 447] products.

The Ins

- Eat plenty (amount dependent on weight, size, sex, and activity level) of whole fruits and vegetables, divided evenly between leafy greens, colored, and sulfur containing.
- Get a high quality blender for easy meals, smoothies, or for gastric feeds. (feedabrain.com/tools)
- Make bone broth and incorporate it into your diet regularly. (feedabrain.com/broth)
  ◊ Get a slow cooker or a pressure cooker to make this much easier. (feedabrain.com/tools)
- Stay adequately hydrated. (feedabrain.com/hydration)
- Heal your gut. (feedabrain.com/digestion)
- Get your blood sugar under control (feedabrain.com/bloodsugar)
- Include adequate, complete proteins (amount dependent on weight, size, sex, and activity level) (feedabrain.com/meat)
- Eat plenty of high-quality fats/oils, cook with the right kinds of fats/oils, and remove bad fats/oils from the diet. (See the Guide to Fats and Oils handout) (feedabrain.com/fat)

- Supply Superfoods (feedabrain.com/superfood).
  - ◊ **Organ meats**
    - The easiest option is to supplement with dessicated organ meat capsules
      (feedabrain.com/ superfood)
    - Get organ meats from feedabrain.com/meat
  - ◊ **Fermented foods**
    - The easiest option is to supplement with probiotics. (feedabrain.com/superfood)
  - ◊ **Sea Vegetables**
    - The easiest option is to alternate between kelp supplements and dulse supplements. (feedabrain.com/superfood)
  - ◊ **Cold Water Fatty Fish (feedabrain.com/fish)**
    - The easiest option is to supplement with one of the fish oils at feedabrain.com/omega
- Supply nutrients for synaptogenesis (feedabrain.com/synapto)
  - ◊ **Choline:**
    - Regularly consume organ meats and/or egg yolks as well as supplemental citicoline. (feedabrain.com/synapto)
  - ◊ **DHA:**
    - Eat cold water fatty fish (feedabrain.com/fish) while also supplementing with recommended fish oils (feedabrain.com/omega)
    - Vegan source of DHA (feedabrain.com/vegan)
    - Supplement with liquid fish oils (feedabrain.com/omega)[448]
  - ◊ **Uridine:**
    - We can get uridine through organ meats, broccoli, beets, and other foods, but we want to also supplement uridine monophosphate (Dr. Wurtman points out that out of the three nutrients for synaptogenesis, uridine is only found in human breast milk, which is not really available to adults.)[449] (feedabrain.com/synapto)

FEEDING A BRAIN FOR REAL

I know that I have a much easier time doing anything after seeing how it's done. This is why I am including many actual meals that I have had. These are captions adapted from my @feedabrain Instagram posts. You can go to feedabrain.com/eats to see what I'm recently eating and, in the comments of a particular dish, you can post your comments and questions. I will also be posting recipes in feedabrain.com/recipes.

- Breakfast at a diner restaurant: All side dishes -- sausage, bacon, mixed veggies, and avocado.
- Lunch at a restaurant: Grilled chicken over a bed of romaine lettuce with tomatoes, pepitas (pumpkin seeds), and corn relish, dressed with olive oil and an herb dressing... and (of course) a side of bacon.
- Dinner: Half of a grass-fed beef hamburger patty and hot wings, but no bun, no ketchup, and no ranch dressing, and served on a bed of greens with onions, tomatoes, avocado, and mustard.
- Breakfast: Wild caught sockeye salmon pan seared with ghee, served with sautéed beet greens, roasted beets, and green onions.
- Lunch: Pasture-raised chicken quarters sautéed with ghee and tarragon, served with sautéed turnip greens, yellow and green onions, green olives, and garlic.
- Dinner is my favorite meal to eat a vegan Feed a Brain style meal (especially after having a meat-heavy breakfast and lunch): Mixed greens (including arugula), fermented ginger beets, fresh tomatoes and scallions, and half an avocado, dressed with olive oil and lemon juice.
- Breakfast without using a cutting board: Smoked salmon on top of mixed greens topped with green onions (cut with scissors) and olive oil. Plus a morning "golden globe latte" made with full fat coconut milk, ghee, mango, and turmeric, blended and topped with a sprinkle of black pepper.
- Lunch Smoothie: Kale and honeydew melon blended with water, mint, and coconut oil.
- Dinner: Wild caught salmon pan seared with ghee, served on a bed of greens topped with grilled asparagus, onions, garlic and basil, surrounded by organic nectarine slices.
- Breakfast: Homemade Texas chili (no beans) over greens with sliced radishes, green onions, avocado, and avocado oil.
- Lunch: Romaine lettuce topped with turkey and pork sausage, roasted beets, fresh onions, and watermelon. Heavily dressed with extra virgin olive oil.
- Fancy "Surf and Surf" Dinner: Tarragon-infused "melt in your mouth" scallops and wild-caught sockeye salmon both pan-seared

with grass-fed ghee, served over a salad of mixed greens and fresh basil with sliced avocado, minced green onions, grape tomatoes, and sautéed sweet yellow onion, dressed with olive oil and a fermented ginger-beet juice.

- Breakfast: Leftover salmon from last night on top of a chopped artisan frisée salad with red onions, capers, and avocado oil.
- Morning beverage: A high-quality protein powder (not soy, whey, or casein powder), dark chocolate (high percentage cacao), avocado oil, and hot water blended and topped with a sprinkle of salt. See feedabrain.com/pantry for good protein powder options.
- Lunch: Green tango lettuce topped with roasted beets and carrots, topped with ground pork and turkey with chopped red onions, sauerkraut from a jar, and green onions.
- Dinner: Wild Alaskan Sockeye Salmon on a bed of kale, Brussels sprouts, broccoli, and green and red cabbage and sautéed with minced garlic, olive oil, and served with sliced white peaches.
- Breakfast: Wild caught canned tuna over mixed greens, topped with a handful of mirepoix (chopped onions, carrots, and celery), dressed with avocado oil.
- Lunch: Feed a Brain tacos -- Chopped al pastor street taco meat (pork) with onions and cilantro, served on collard green leaves instead of tortilla.
- Lunch coffee: decaf coffee blended with avocado oil until creamy and sprinkled with a dash of cinnamon.
- Dinner Smoothie: mixed frozen berries, mixed greens, and full fat coconut milk.

A FINAL WORD FROM CAVIN

I hope you've enjoyed this book as much as I loved writing it. I can't tell you how much it means to me to be able to share these tools and to move forward with my mission to pay my fortune forward by sharing what I have found to be especially helpful.

Progress Not Perfection

I know that implementing these changes is not exactly easy. As I studied after my injury, I could see that I absolutely needed to make these dietary changes if I were to give my brain the best shot at recovery. Perhaps you are in that place now. I created this book to be the guide and resource that I wish I had. Knowing what will support neurological recovery can help us to make incremental changes towards better brain health. This is not about perfection. I don't get all of my fruits and veggies every single day, but I try to get close. I didn't start on the sea vegetables or organ meats for years, and I'm not perfect with my supplementation and nutrient intake. I never gave up when I slipped, and I have found some pretty cool tricks to supply these nutrients regularly.

Remember that the bottom line is this:

The healthiest thing we can do for our brains, bodies, and souls is to enjoy our life and to do so sustainably.

You now have the tools to build something life-changing.

If you have an extra minute, I would love to hear what you think about this book. Please leave a review on Amazon.com and if you'd rather reach out in private, you can contact us at feedabrain.com/contact. We try to read each and every comment and email, so come and say hi! You can find more free content on FeedaBrain.com, the Adventures in Brain Injury Podcast, and on YouTube. If you haven't already, you can follow me on Twitter, Instagram, Pinterest (@feedabrain and @cavinb), and like the Feed a Brain Facebook Page. Thanks again, and I wish you the best of health, recovery, and success.

FAQ

Q: How do I handle intense cravings?
A: Inflammatory foods trigger an immune response, causing certain neurotransmitters, such as adrenaline, to be secreted. The brain can become addicted to the rush of adrenaline caused by this immune response, essentially creating an addiction to the inflammatory food *because* it is inflammatory.[450] At the same time, the brain and body are going through a mini-crisis while trying to figure out how to transition metabolism to this neuroprotective way of eating.

The most common intense craving is for sugar and starches like pasta, bread, desserts, donuts, cookies, or candies. The brain and body's metabolism is craving energy while switching from a fuel source of sugar and carbs to the brain's more efficient and neuroprotective fuel: fat. The easiest way to bypass these cravings is by introducing exogenous ketones while following the "Feed a Brain" guidelines. Go to feedabrain.com/keto for information on how to Feed a Brain keto style.

These are some other methods which may be helpful:
Eat some protein and fat every two hours. Add whole fruits and/or roasted vegetables as desired.

Keep non-starchy vegetables ready to eat so that you can calm sugar cravings. See the Batch Cooking Handout.

L-Glutamine, an amino acid involved in fat metabolism that is also an excellent support to heal leaky gut and/or cinnamon mixed with water makes a great elixir to calm down the craving even further.

Because of the difficulty involved in this transition, you can also have good choices like a sweet potato or a piece of fruit, while supplying good fat (like ghee) to encourage the metabolism to switch over. You can get more information on this at feedabrain.com/bloodsugar. Again, the easiest way to facilitate this transition is to introduce exogenous ketones while still eating a high fat/low carb diet. Go to feedabrain.com/keto for more information about exogenous ketones.

Q: If I forget to take my supplements, should I take them with my next supplements?

A: No. Just try not to miss them in the future. We don't want to overwhelm our system by taking too much at one time.

Q: I don't have time to prepare these meals. Can I get these foods pre-made?

A: We are working on making pre-made meals available for delivery. Visit feedabrain.com/premade.

Q: How important is it for me to eliminate wheat?

A: Cutting wheat is what Dr. Datis Kharrazian says is the most effective practice that you can do for your brain health.[451] The gluten found in wheat is not what it was even 50 years ago.[452, 453] Today's wheat is clearly not fatal, but even a tiny bit can cause an immune response that likely inflames the brain.

Act as if you have celiac disease for at least 60 days. Shop for only sauces that are labeled gluten free, and ask restaurants for gluten free options. Cross-contamination should be avoided as well. The strictness of this rule will likely not be forever. Go to feedabrain.com/gluten for more information and support.

Q: Can I get all of the beneficial minerals from broth in a box or can?

A: Unfortunately, the short answer is no. Many health experts agree that when a broth is made the traditional way (from bones), it contains so many more minerals and nutrients that are lost through the sterilization and aseptic packaging of store-bought broths.[454 455] What is done to make the store-bought broth shelf stable may degrade certain compounds in the broth that make many of the nutrients bioavailable. Bioavailability is the amount that a nutrient is usable by, or available to, our bodies. When we lose what makes these nutrients bioavailable, many of the vitamins, minerals, collagen, gelatin, and other nutrients in the broth are no longer usable by our brains or bodies.[456] While you can still use boxed, canned, or powdered bone broth, you will not get all of the beneficial nutrients that are found in homemade broth. Go to feedabrain.com/broth for more options and information.

Q: When should I start?
A: The most effective way is to jump into it as soon as you can. Procrastinating seems to make it so much harder to follow. It gives your mind the time to talk yourself out of it. We humans resist change. We even resist change when our current behavior is not working for us. If you have ever been or known someone in a toxic relationship, you have witnessed this phenomenon. It is the basis of addiction, battered person syndrome, and the like. Because of the fear of the unknown and the comfort of familiarity, we resist change until the pain of the problem is worse than the pain of the solution. Most people would rather stay in a place that they know is not working than to try something new. Don't be like most people. Dive in and change your life today! I am building classes and I also work one-on-one with clients. Go to feedabrain.com/consult or feedabrain.com/education.

Q: How will I stick to this?
A: We have a choice of what our mindset will be during this time. Our perspectives can either be of deprivation or abundance. This is not about deprivation; this is about removing the foods that could be harming us and ramping up the foods that fuel the cells of our brains and bodies. To use our analogy from earlier, this is about not slamming our thumb in the drawer while tending to the wounds.

When I first embarked on this way of eating, it helped me to remember that I had been through so much worse than the potentially uncomfortable changes that I would experience. Many other survivors can relate to this perspective and have been able to use it to stick to this program. My brain and body needed a rest from what it had endured and the foods that did not support its function, while it obtained all the nutrients that did. Exogenous ketones can really take the edge off as well. Go to feedabrain.com/keto for more information on exogenous ketones.

Q: Allergy testing has shown that I don't (or my loved one doesn't) have an immune response to _____. Should I still remove this food?

A: If it is a food that is outlined to be avoided or removed in this meal plan, then the answer is yes, I think you should still remove it. Why? Because standard allergy testing does not address all types of immune responses that a person may have to a specific food. There are different immune response systems within our bodies which have specific types of antibodies associated with them. Most commonly-ordered allergy testing only tests one of these systems, not all of them at once, which is what would be necessary to effectively rule out an immune reaction to foods. Therefore, on a test that screens for one type of antibodies, you may test negative, but still be having an immune response that the test does not screen for. Because of this, allergy testing can often result in a false negative stating there is no immune reaction, when there is actually one present. For this reason, traditional allergy testing is not a reliable way to truly know what foods are problematic for you, so an elimination diet is preferred.[457]

The gold standard of an elimination diet is used by many functional practitioners. This takes some time and effort from the patient. Here's how it's done:

1. The food needs to be removed 100% for at least 30 days, but it may take up to 90 days for any possible immune response to subside (this guide suggests 60 days).

2. The next step is to reintroduce the food in a substantial amount for a few days and to observe any possible changes in feeling, mucus or saliva secretion, trouble breathing, brain function, anxiety, temper, pain, digestive symptoms, or any other change that occurs, even if seemingly unrelated. An immune response can show itself in an infinite number of possible responses.

3. If you notice an effect throughout this experiment, the food likely creates an inflammatory response at that time. Try waiting 30 days more than the last removal period and try again (immune reactions can sometimes subside), or simply remove the food from your diet. I still recommend removing both wheat and milk because of the above studies.

It takes some detective work to eliminate potentially inflammatory foods 100%. We also need to pay attention to the ingredients of sauces, toothpastes, deodorants, soaps, skincare, etc. Wheat and milk containing products are found in many places that most of us never think about.

Double check these kinds of products for inflammatory compounds (all products found on feedabrain.com are free of gluten, harmful proteins found in dairy, and egg):

- Sunscreens and lotions.
- Shampoos, conditioners, cosmetics, and styling products.
- Lip balm and glosses.
- Spices, salad dressing, dip, and soup mixes.
- Imitation crab (may include eggs and/or gluten).
- Beer (most beer is made with wheat, yeast, rye, oats, and/or barley).
- Worcestershire, soy, BBQ, and other sauces.
- Play Dough (may be made with wheat flour
- Vitamins, supplements, and medication[458]

Q: Why is it that consumption of ghee (clarified butter) is encouraged when ghee is made from milk?
A: While ghee is made from milk, by clarifying it, only trace amounts of milk proteins (e.g. casein) and lactose are left in ghee, and it is well tolerated by almost all. Additionally, ghee contains extremely beneficial fatty acids like CLA, and the process of clarifying butter is easy and natural. In fact, all you need to do to clarify your own butter is to melt it and to pour it through 3 or more layers of cheesecloth.

Q: What about a little cheat? Why are there no cheat days?
A: We cannot really cheat on all of the things that we want to add to our diet. We can only fall short. And if we fall short one day, we can do a little better the next day. We can, however, cheat by going overboard on foods that we want to avoid, but in doing so, we are cheating ourselves.

If we are eating the six to nine fists of produce, plenty of healthy fats, sea vegetables, fermented foods, organ meats, and cold water fatty fish, while also supplying the three nutrients for synaptogenesis, there likely won't be room for many of the foods that we want to avoid. But, for motivation's sake, I tell myself that I can have any of the foods that I know do not serve me, but only *after* I include everything else that is important for my brain health.

The other way we might cheat is by eating foods that we have decided to remove during a 60-day elimination diet. For us to see the effects of inflammatory foods, we need to eliminate them 100% for at least 60 days. When we are already experiencing significant inflammation, we are unable to perceive a new inflammatory response. Again, how can one tell that it's raining when underwater? This really is not the time to cheat. Bite the bullet and stick to it.

If you do cheat before going 60 consecutive days without any exposure to these foods, don't give up. It's okay. We are all human, and we are going to slip up from time to time. We can try again and make progress, and one day we will make it 60 days without any exposure to the food. We can then reintroduce it to determine if we really want to include it in our diet. After taking these important steps to see what we can do to best support our brain health, we can allow ourselves a "cheat" by exposing ourselves to small amounts of a food that we know is inflammatory. But like I said, if we cheat before 60 days, we are only cheating ourselves of knowing whether or not a food supports the health of our brains and bodies.

Q: What if I don't like to cook?

A: I hear you. I mean, I like to cook, but not when I *have* to cook. Coming up with food choices should not be stressful. In fact, studies have shown that digestion is impaired by stress.[459] Whether at home or on the go, try to be prepared with brain building nourishment that can be ready immediately or in a few minutes when you can't, or don't feel like cooking. We are also working to arrange for the availability of pre-made Feed a Brain approved meals that can be delivered to your door and then simply heated before eating. Go to feedabrain.com/premade.

Q: Why does my loved one (or I) have no appetite? How can I get them (or myself) to consume all of these brain building nutrients?

A: The sympathetic, or "fight or flight," nervous system kicks into high gear during trauma or fear. This is the nervous system that takes over when someone needs to run from danger. When the sympathetic, or "fight or flight," nervous system is dominant, digestion and obtaining nutrients move way down on the priority list, and instead, the focus is put on escaping the danger, even if doing so is at the expense of health. [460, 461]

The thing is, the nervous system doesn't know the difference between being chased by a lion or hearing something that upsets it. What we can do to help move someone out of this fight or flight state is to help them to feel safe and to experience less stress. While finding ways to reduce your loved one's stress, an excellent strategy to help supply these nutrients is with nutrient-dense beverages. Not always, but often times when someone does not have an appetite, they still experience thirst.

A rich, high-quality bone broth or Feed a Brain smoothie is a great start. Adding a tasty combination of vegetables, fruits, and good fats to be blended using a Vitamix™ or Blendtec™ has also been effective. You can combine a soup with a nutrient-dense smoothie with all three categories of produce in roughly equal amounts, adequate fat and protein, along with some super foods, and the nutrients for synaptogenesis found at feedabrain.com/synapto.

Q: How do I approach the hospital to request a dietary change?
A: As described in the Considerations of a Blenderized Gastric Diet section, when requesting a dietary change from the healthcare team, we first need to create a relationship that can hopefully evolve into a partnership for the patient's well-being. Always approach them with compassion and a desire to help them to help your loved one. After all, at the end of the day, you both share the same goal: for the patient to get better. Be friendly, empathetic, and confident when speaking with people on the healthcare team. Express to them why your loved one matters to you. After your humanity, pain, and confidence have been relayed, bring up this guide, tell them what you have learned, and tell them what you would like to do for your loved one and why. Show that you are willing to put in the effort and ask them if they will help. You may need to order the gastric feeds and have them delivered every day, but food is medicine, and this is how we can feed the cells in our brains and bodies. As Dr. Terry Wahls says, "When we take care of our cells, our cells take care of us."

ADDITIONAL RESOURCES & TIPS

- **Get blood sugar support:**
  - ◊ Sweet Tooth Bitter Truth – feedabrain.com/bloodsugar
- **Absorb Your Nutrients. Heal Your Gut:**
  - ◊ Solving Leaky Gut - feedabrain.com/digestion
- **Order Quality Food**
  - ◊ **Pre-made Meals** - feedabrain.com/premade
  - ◊ **High Quality Fish**- feedabrain.com/fish
  - ◊ **High Quality Meats** - feedabrain.com/meat
  - ◊ **Pantry foods** - feedabrain.com/pantry
- **Gastric Feeds**
  - ◊ **Feed a Brain Approved Gastric Feeds** – feedabrain.com/feeds
  - ◊ **Pre-made Meals + Bone Broth for Blending** – feedabrain.com/premade
  - ◊ **Blenders for Blenderized Tube Feeds** – feedabrain.com/tools
- **Supplements**–feedabrain.com/supplements
  - ◊ **Nutrients for Synaptogenesis** – feedabrain.com/synapto
  - ◊ **To Support Brain Metabolism** – feedabrain.com/atp
  - ◊ **To Reduce Brain Inflammation** – feedabrain.com/ros
- **Food on The Go:**
  - ◊ Carry a cooler with smoothies, soups, salads, and/or unsweetened coconut yogurt
  - ◊ Stay hydrated. I love this water bottle because it is entirely spill proof: feedabrain.com/hydration
  - ◊ Grass-Fed jerky or meat bars – feedabrain.com/meat or canned fish – feedabrain.com/fish
  - ◊ Sunflower seeds, pumpkin seeds, and pine nuts
  - ◊ Carrots, celery, broccoli, peppers, and cauliflower in plastic baggies
  - ◊ Dehydrated organic veggies
  - ◊ Carry fruit from the colored list (oranges, plums, peaches, berries)

CITATION NOTES

¹ National Institute of Mental Health. "Any Mental Illness (AMI) Among U.S. Adults." Accessed October 1, 2017. https://www.nimh.nih.gov/health/statistics/prevalence/any-mental-illness-ami-among-us-adults.shtml.

² Lundy-Ekman, Laurie. *Neuroscience: Fundamentals for Rehabilitation (3rd ed.)* (St. Louis: Saunders Elsevier Inc., 2007), 28-29.

³ Mason, Peggy. *Medical Neurobiology* (New York: Oxford University Press, 2011), 4.

⁴ Doidge, Norman. *The Brain That Changes Itself: Stories of Personal Triumph from the Frontiers of Brain Science.* (New York: Penguin Books, 2007), xvii-xix, 12-13.

⁵ Schwartz, Jeffrey M. and Sharon Begley. *The Mind & The Brain: Neuroplasticity and the Power of Mental Energy.* (New York: Harper Collins Publishers, Inc., 2003), chapter 1.

⁶ Doidge, Norman. *The Brain That Changes Itself*, xvii-xix, 12-13.

⁷ Ramachandran, V.S. preface to *The Tell-Tale Brain: A Neuroscientist's Quest for What Makes Us Human* (New York: W. W. Norton & Company, Inc., 2011), xiii.

⁸ Doidge, Norman. Book description for *The Brain That Changes Itself.* Available at https://www.penguinrandomhouse.com/books/291041/the-brain-that-changes-itself-by-norman-doidge/9780670038305/.

[9] Grant, Gunnar. "How the 1906 Nobel Prize in physiology or medicine was shared between Golgi and Cajal," *Brain Research Reviews* 55.2 (2007): 490-98.

[10] Schwartz, Jeffrey M. and Sharon Begley. *The Mind & The Brain,* chapter 1.

[11] Schwartz, Jeffrey M. and Sharon Begley. *The Mind & The Brain,* chapter 1.

[12] Lundy-Ekman, Laurie. *Neuroscience: Fundamentals for Rehabilitation,* 71-83.

[13] Lundy-Ekman, Laurie. *Neuroscience: Fundamentals for Rehabilitation,* 4.

[14] Lundy-Ekman, Laurie. *Neuroscience: Fundamentals for Rehabilitation,* 4-14.

[15] Lundy-Ekman, Laurie. *Neuroscience: Fundamentals for Rehabilitation,* 28-30.

[16] Lundy-Ekman, Laurie. *Neuroscience: Fundamentals for Rehabilitation,* 28-30.

[17] Lundy-Ekman, Laurie. *Neuroscience: Fundamentals for Rehabilitation,* 39-42, 47.

[18] Gómez-Pinilla, Fernando. "Brain foods: the effects of nutrients on brain function," *Nature Reviews Neuroscience* 9.7 (2008): 568-578.

[19] Bender, David A. I*ntroduction to Nutrition and Metabolism* (5th ed.) (Boca Raton,FL: CRC Press, 2014), 1-4.

[20] Bender, David A. *Introduction to Nutrition and Metabolism,* 1-4.

[21] Sherwood, Lauralee. *Human Physiology: From Cells to Systems* (9th ed.) (Boston: Cengage Learning, 2015), 566-72.

[22] Drubach, Daniel. *The Brain Explained* (Upper Saddle River, NJ: Prentice Hall, 2000).

[23] Brown, Guy. *The Energy of Life: The Science of What Makes Our Minds and Bodies Work* (New York: The Free Press, 1999).

24 Hart, Leslie A. *How the Brain Works: A New Understanding of Human Learning, Emotion, and Thinking* (New York: Basic Books,1975).

25 Wurtman, Richard J. and Judith J Wurtman. *Nutrition and the Brain. Volume 2. Control of feeding behavior and biology of the brain in protein-calorie malnutrition* (New York: Raven Press, 1977).

26 Youdim, Kuresh A. and James A Joseph. "A possible emerging role of phytochemicals in improving age-related neurological dysfunctions: a multiplicity of effects," *Free Radical Biology and Medicine* 30.6 (2001): 583-94.

27 Azevedo, Frederico A.C., et. al. "Equal Numbers of Neuronal and Nonneuronal Cells Make the Human Brain an Isometrically Scaled-Up Primate Brain," *The Journal of Comparative Neurology* 513 (2009):532–41. doi 10.1002/cne.21974.

28 Azevedo, Frederico A.C., et. al. "Equal Numbers of Neuronal and Nonneuronal Cells Make the Human Brain an Isometrically Scaled-Up Primate Brain" 532–41.

29 Lundy-Ekman, Laurie. *Neuroscience: Fundamentals for Rehabilitation*, 43-46.

30 Lundy-Ekman, Laurie. *Neuroscience: Fundamentals for Rehabilitation*, 44 .

31 Johnson, Victoria E., William Stewart, Douglas H.Smith. "Axonal pathology in traumatic brain injury," *Experimental Neurology* 246 (August 2013): 35-43. Available online January 20, 2012. doi.org/10.1016/j.expneurol.2012.01.013

32 Johnson, Victoria E., William Stewart, Douglas H.Smith.. "Widespread Tau and Amyloid-Beta Pathology Many Years After a Single Traumatic Brain Injury in Humans," *Brain Pathology* 22 (2) (March 2012): 142-49. doi/10.1111/j.1750-3639.2011.00513.x.

33 Masliah E , et al. "Cortical dendritic pathology in human immunodeficiency virus encephalitis," *Laboratory Investigation; a Journal of Technical Methods and Pathology* 66(3) (01 Mar 1992): 285-91. http://europepmc.org/abstract/med/1538584

34 "Wikipedia "Organism" (12 Apr. 2016) Available at https://en.wikipedia. org/wiki/Organism, accessed on October 2, 2017.

35 Koshland, Daniel E. "The Seven Pillars of Life," *Science* 295.5563 (2002): 2215-216.

36 Mayer, Emeran A. "Gut feelings: the emerging biology of gut–brain communication," *Nature Reviews Neuroscience* 12.8 (2011): 453-66.

37 Kharrazian, Datis. *Why Isn't My Brain Working?: A revolutionary understanding of brain decline and effective strategies to recover your brain health* (Carlsbad, CA: Elephant Press, 2013), 163-66.

38 Furness, John Barton, and Marcelo Costa. "Types of nerves in the enteric nervous system." *Neuroscience* 5.1 (1980): 1-20.

39 Furness, John Barton and Marcelo Costa. *The Enteric Nervous System.* (London: Churchill Livingstone, 1987).

40 Permlutter, David E. *Grain Brain: The Surprising Truth About Wheat, Carbs, and Sugar—Your Brain's Silent Killers* (New York: Little, Brown and Company, 2013), 190.

41 Gershon, Michael MD. *The Second Brain: The Scientific Basis of Gut Instinct and a Groundbreaking New Understanding of Nervous Disorders of the Stomach and Intestines* (New York: Harper, 1998).

42 Kim, Doe-Young, and Michael Camilleri. "Serotonin: a mediator of the brain-gut connection," *The American Journal of Gastroenterology* 95.10 (2000): 2698.

43 Martin, MT, F Azpiroz, and JR Malagelada. "Melatonin and the gastrointestinal tract," *Thérapie* 53.5 (1997): 453-58.

44 Messner, Michael et al. "Presence of melatonin in the human hepatobiliary-gastrointestinal tract," *Life Sciences* 69.5 (2001): 543-51.

[45] Kim, Doe-Young and Michael Camilleri. "Serotonin: a mediator of the brain-gut connection" 2698.

[46] Martin, MT, F Azpiroz, and JR Malagelada. "Melatonin and the gastrointestinal tract." 453-58.

[47] Messner, Michael et al. "Presence of melatonin in the human hepatobiliary-gastrointestinal tract" 543-51.

[48] Permutter, David E. *Grain Brain*, 178-81.

[49] Bansal, Vishal et al. "Traumatic brain injury and intestinal dysfunction: uncovering the neuro-enteric axis," *Journal of Neurotrauma* 26.8 (2009): 1353-359.

[50] Forsyth, Christopher B et al. "Increased intestinal permeability correlates with sigmoid mucosa alpha-synuclein staining and endotoxin exposure markers in early Parkinson's disease," *PLOS ONE* 6.12 (2011): e28032.

[51] Mass, Michael, Marta Kubera, and Jean-Claude Leunis. "The gut-brain barrier in major depression: intestinal mucosal dysfunction with an increased translocation of LPS from gram negative enterobacteria (leaky gut) plays a role in the inflammatory pathophysiology of depression," *Neuroendocrinology Letters* 29.1 (2008): 117-24.

[52] Bansal, Vishal et al. "Traumatic brain injury and intestinal dysfunction: uncovering the neuro-enteric axis" 1353-359.

[53] Forsyth, Christopher B et al. "Increased intestinal permeability correlates with sigmoid mucosa alpha-synuclein staining and endotoxin exposure markers in early Parkinson's disease." *PLOS ONE* 6.12 (2011): e28032.

[54] Petra, Anastasia, et al. "Gut-Microbiota-Brain Axis and its Effect on Neuropsychiatric Disorders with Suspected Immune Dysregulation," *Clinical Therapeutics* 37 (2015): 984-995

55 Dunlop, Simon, et al. "Abnormal Intestinal Permeability in Subgroups of Diarrhea-Predominant Irritable Bowel Syndromes," *The American Journal of Gastroenterology* 101 (2006):1288-294.

56 Jackson, P.G, et al. "Intestinal Permeability In Patients With Eczema And Food Allergy," *The Lancet* (1981): 1285-286.

57 Jenkins, R., et al. "Increased Intestinal Permeability In Patients With Rheumatoid Arthritis: A Side-Effect Of Oral Nonsteroidal Anti-Inflammatory Drug Therapy?," *Rheumatology* (1987): 103-07.

58 Visser, Jeroen, et al. "Tight Junctions, Intestinal Permeability, and Autoimmunity," *Annals of the New York Academy of Sciences* (2009): 195-205

59 Fasano, Alessio. "Zonulin and Its Regulation of Intestinal Barrier Function: The biological Door to Inflammation, Autoimmunity, and Cancer," *Physiological Reviews* 91.1 (2011): 151-75.

60 Arrieta MC, Bistritz L, Meddings JB. "Alterations in intestinal permeability," *Gut* 55 (2006):1512-520.

61 Fasano, Alessio and Terez Shea-Donohue. "Mechanisms of Disease: the role of intestinal barrier function in the pathogenesis of gastrointestinal autoimmune diseases." *Gastroenterology and Hepatology* 2 (September 2005): 416-22. doi:10.1038/ncpgasthep0259.

62 Kharrazian, Datis. *Why Isn't My Brain Working?*, 175-77.

63 Sherwood, Lauralee. *Human Physiology*, 566-72.

64 Arrieta MC, et al. "Alterations in Intestinal Permeability"1512-520.

65 Fasano, Alessio and Terez Shea-Donohue. "Mechanisms of Disease: the role of intestinal barrier function in the pathogenesis of gastrointestinal autoimmune diseases" 416-22.

66 Arrieta MC, et al. "Alterations in intestinal permeability" 1512-520.

[67] Fasano, Alessio and Terez Shea-Donohue. "Mechanisms of Disease: the role of intestinal barrier function in the pathogenesis of gastrointestinal autoimmune diseases" 416-22.

[68] Arrieta MC, et al. "Alterations in intestinal permeability" 1512-520.

[69] Fasano, Alessio and Terez Shea-Donohue. "Mechanisms of Disease: the role of intestinal barrier function in the pathogenesis of gastrointestinal autoimmune diseases" 416-22.

[70] Kharrazian, Datis. *Why Isn't My Brain Working?*, 175-77.

[71] Wahls, Terry L. *The Wahls Protocol: A Radical New Way to Treat All Chronic Autoimmune Conditions Using Paleo Principles* (New York: Avery, 2014), 91.

[72] Lundy-Ekman, Laurie. *Neuroscience: Fundamentals for Rehabilitation,* 495-97.

[73] Wahls, Terry L. *The Wahls Protocol,* 91.

[74] Kharrazian, Datis. *Why Isn't My Brain Working?,* 204-208.

[75] Banks, WA, AJ Kastin, and RD Broadwell. "Passage of cytokines across the blood-brain barrier," *Neuroimmunomodulation* 2.4 (1995): 241-48.

[76] Banks, WA, AJ Kastin, and RD Broadwell. "Passage of cytokines across the blood-brain barrier" 241-48.

[77] Kharrazian, Datis. *Why Isn't My Brain Working?,* 199-200.

[78] Ekdahl, Christine T. et al. "Inflammation is detrimental for neurogenesis in adult brain," *Proceedings of the National Academy of Sciences* 100.23 (2003): 13632-3637.

[79] Nimmo, AJ et al. "Neurogenic inflammation is associated with development of edema and functional deficits following traumatic brain injury in rats," *Neuropeptides* 38.1 (2004): 40-47.

⁸⁰ Moore, TC. "Modification of lymphocyte traffic by vasoactive neurotransmitter substances," *Immunology* 52.3 (1984): 511.

⁸¹ Swank, Gregory M. and Edwin A Deitch. "Role of the gut in multiple organ failure: bacterial translocation and permeability changes," *World Journal of Surgery* 20.4 (1996): 411-17.

⁸² Kharrazian, Datis. *Why Isn't My Brain Working?*, 42-43, 101-02.

⁸³ Swank, Gregory M. and Edwin A Deitch. "Role of the gut in multiple organ failure: bacterial translocation and permeability changes" 411-17.

⁸⁴Nimmo, AJ et al. "Neurogenic inflammation is associated with development of edema and functional deficits following traumatic brain injury in rats," *Neuropeptides* 38.1 (2004): 40-47.

⁸⁵ Banks, WA, AJ Kastin, and RD Broadwell. "Passage of cytokines across the blood-brain barrier" 241-48.

⁸⁶ Perlmutter, David E. *Grain Brain*, 61-62.

⁸⁷ Kharrazian, Datis. *Why Isn't My Brain Working?*, 36, 38, 42-43, 101-102, 175.

⁸⁸ Perlmutter, David E. *Grain Brain*, 33, 61-62.

⁸⁹ Kharrazian, Datis. *Why Isn't My Brain Working?*, 36, 38, 175.

⁹⁰ Perlmutter, David E. *Grain Brain*, 33, 51, 53, 61-62.

⁹¹ Dr. Tom O'Bryan has stated this in many interviews, articles, presentations, and podcasts. One example is available at: http://thedr.com/wp-content/uploads/2014/07/Top-3-Tips_Edit_073014.pd (accessed on September 25, 2017).

⁹² O'Bryan, Tom. *The Autoimmune Fix* (New York: Rodale Inc., 2015), 59 (quoting Alessio Fasano, MD, "The state of health or the state of disease is the

combination between what we are—meaning what genetically makes us the way that we're engineered—and the environment that's around us. And the gut is the point of entry in which these two elements meet.").

[93] Cryan, John F. and Timothy G. Dinan. "Mind-altering microorganisms: the impact of the gut microbiota on brain and behaviour." *Nature Reviews Neuroscience* 13 (October 2012): 701-12. doi:10.1038/nrn3346

[94] Alberts, B., et al. "How Cells Obtain Energy from Food" *Molecular Biology of the Cell*. 4th ed. (New York: Garland Science; 2002). Available at https://www.ncbi.nlm.nih.gov/books/NBK26882/.

[95] Sherwood, Lauralee. *Human Physiology*, 33-40.

[96] Fiebich BL, S Akter and RS Akundi. "The two-hit hypothesis for neuroinflammation: role of exogenous ATP in modulating inflammation in the brain," *Front. Cell. Neurosci.* 8 (2014):260. doi: 10.3389/fncel.2014.00260

[97] Sherwood, Lauralee. *Human Physiology*, 33-40.

[98] Kharrazian, Datis. *Why Isn't My Brain Working?*, 119 ("ATP is the fuel source for all biochemical reactions.")

[99] https://en.oxforddictionaries.com/definition/nutrient

[100] Sherwood, Lauralee. *Human Physiology*, 33-40.

[101] Ames Bruce N. "Micronutrients prevent cancer and delay aging," *Toxicology Letters* 102–103 (28 December 1998): 5-18. https://doi.org/10.1016/S0378-4274(98)00269-0

[102] Ames Bruce N. "Micronutrients prevent cancer and delay aging" 5-18.

[103] Cassidy, A. and C. D. Kay. "Phytochemicals" Chapter in *Nutrition and Metabolism* 2nd ed. (eds S. A. Lanham-New, I. A. Macdonald and H. M. Roche) (Oxford, UK: Wiley-Blackwell, 2010), chapter 14. doi: 10.1002/9781444327779.ch14.

[104] Wahls, Terry L. *The Wahls Protocol.*

[105] Vercellino, Marco et al. "Grey Matter Pathology in Multiple Sclerosis," *Journal of Neuropathology & Experimental Neurology* 64 (12) (1 December 2005): 1101–107. doi.org/10.1097/01.jnen.0000190067.20935.42

[106] Wahls, Terry L. *The Wahls Protocol,* 7.

[107] Wahls, Terry L. *The Wahls Protocol,* 9-10.

[108] See the website of the Institute for Functional Medicine available at https://www.ifm.org/functional-medicine/.

[109] https://www.ifm.org/functional-medicine/

[110] Wahls, Terry L. *The Wahls Protocol,* 9-10.

[111] Wahls, Terry L. *The Wahls Protocol,* 9-10.

[112] Berkow, Susan, and Sushma Palmer. "Nutrition in medical education: current status and future directions." *The Journal of Nutrition* 116.3 (1986): 341-342.

[113] Minger, Denise. *Death by Food Pyramid.* Primal Blueprint Publishing, 2013.

[114] Wahls, Terry L. *The Wahls Protocol,* 8.

[115] Wahls, Terry L. *The Wahls Protocol,* 11.

[116] Wahls, Terry L. *The Wahls Protocol,* 11.

[117] Bender, David A. *Introduction to Nutrition and Metabolism,* 1-6.

[118] Wahls, Terry L. *The Wahls Protocol,* 11.

[119] Wahls, Terry L. *The Wahls Protocol,* 11.

[120] Wahls, Terry L. *The Wahls Protocol*, 11.

[121] Wahls, Terry L. *The Wahls Protocol*, 12.

[122] http://terrywahls.com/about/about-terry-wahls/

[123] Wahls, Terry L. *The Wahls Protocol*.

[124] Kharrazian, Datis. *Why Isn't My Brain Working?*, 199-200.

[125] Wahls, Terry L. *The Wahls Protocol*.

[126] Perlmutter, David E. *Grain Brain*, 70-84.

[127] Nierenberg, Danielle. "Factory farming in The Developing World," *World Watch* 16.3 (2003): 10-19.

[128] Herrmann, Wolfgang, et al. "Vitamin B-12 status, particularly holotranscobalamin II and methylmalonic acid concentrations, and hyperhomocysteinemia in vegetarians., *The American Journal of Clinical Nutrition* 78.1 (2003): 131-36.

[129] Rosell, Magdalena S et al. "Long-chain n–3 polyunsaturated fatty acids in plasma in British meat-eating, vegetarian, and vegan men," *The American Journal of Clinical Nutrition* 82.2 (2005): 327-334.

[130] Dwyer, Johanna T. "Nutritional Consequences of Vegetarianism," *Annual Review of Nutrition* 11.1 (1991): 61-91.

[131] Hunt, Janet R. "Bioavailability of iron, zinc, and other trace minerals from vegetarian diets," *The American Journal of Clinical Nutrition* 78.3 (2003): 633S-639S.

[132] Bailes, Julian E. and James D Mills. "Docosahexaenoic acid reduces traumatic axonal injury in a rodent head injury model," *Journal of Neurotrauma* 27.9 (2010): 1617-624.

[133] Mills, James D et al. "Omega-3 fatty acid supplementation and reduction of traumatic axonal injury in a rodent head injury model: Laboratory investigation," *Journal of Neurosurgery* 114.1 (2011): 77-84.

[134] Lewis, Michael, Parviz Ghassemi and Joseph Hibbeln. "Therapeutic use of omega-3 fatty acids in severe head trauma," *The American Journal of Emergency Medicine* 31.1 (2013): 273. e5-273. e8.

[135] Lewis, Michael, et al. "Therapeutic use of omega-3 fatty acids in severe head trauma" 273. e5-273. e8.

[136] Lewis, Michael, et al. "Therapeutic use of omega-3 fatty acids in severe head trauma" 273. e5-273. e8.

[137] Damude, Howard G. and Anthony J Kinney. "Engineering oilseed plants for a sustainable, land-based source of long chain polyunsaturated fatty acids," *Lipids* 42.3 (2007): 179-185.

[138] Haggarty, P et al. "Long-chain polyunsaturated fatty acid transport across the perfused human placenta," *Placenta* 18.8 (1997): 635-642.

[139] Gerster, H. "Can adults adequately convert alpha-linolenic acid (18: 3n-3) to eicosapentaenoic acid (20: 5n-3) and docosahexaenoic acid (22: 6n-3)?," *International Journal for Vitamin and Nutrition Research. Internationale Zeitschrift für Vitamin-und Ernährungsforschung. Journal International de Vitaminologie et de Nutrition* 68.3 (1997): 159-173.

[140] Arterburn, Linda M et al. "Bioequivalence of docosahexaenoic acid from different algal oils in capsules and in a DHA-fortified food," *Lipids* 42.11 (2007): 1011-024.

[141] Doughman, Scott D, Srirama Krupanidhi, and Carani B Sanjeevi. "Omega-3 fatty acids for nutrition and medicine: considering microalgae oil as a vegetarian source of EPA and DHA," *Current Diabetes Reviews* 3.3 (2007): 198-203.

[142] Conquer, Julie A. and Bruce J Holub. "Supplementation with an algae source of docosahexaenoic acid increases (n-3) fatty acid status and alters

selected risk factors for heart disease in vegetarian subjects," *The Journal of Nutrition* 126.12 (1996): 3032.

[143] Spruss, Astrid and Ina Bergheim. "Dietary fructose and intestinal barrier: potential risk factor in the pathogenesis of nonalcoholic fatty liver disease," *The Journal of Nutritional Biochemistry* 20.9 (2009): 657-662.

[144] Gibson, PR, and SJ Shepherd. "Personal view: food for thought–western lifestyle and susceptibility to Crohn's disease. The FODMAP hypothesis," *Alimentary Pharmacology & Therapeutics* 21.12 (2005): 1399-409.

[145] Csáki, Katalin F. "Synthetic surfactant food additives can cause intestinal barrier dysfunction," *Medical Hypotheses* 76.5 (2011): 676-81.

[146] Akoh, Casimir C. and David B Min. *Food Lipids: Chemistry, Nutrition, and Biotechnology* (Boca Raton: CRC press, 2008).

[147] Rose, GA, WB Thomson, and RT Williams. "Corn oil in treatment of ischaemic heart disease," *British Medical Journal* 1.5449 (1965): 1531.

[148] Moret, Sabrina, A Dudine, and LS Conte. "Processing effects on the polyaromatic hydrocarbon content of grapeseed oil," *Journal of the American Oil Chemists' Society* 77.12 (2000): 1289-292.

[149] Body Nutrition. "Grapeseed Oil provides minimal benefits, lacks nutrients." Retrieved September 10, 2017, from https://bodynutrition.org/grapeseed-oil/.

[150] Smith, J. M. "Are Genetically Modified Foods a Gut-Wrenching Combination?" Responsible Technology. Retrieved September 10, 2017, from http://responsibletechnology.org/glutenintroduction/

[151] Kharrazian, Datis, *Why Isn't My Brain Working?*, 36, 38, 42-43, 101-102, 175.

[152] Perlmutter, David E. *Grain Brain*, 51, 53, 61-62.

153 Daulatzai, Mak A. "Non-Celiac Gluten Sensitivity Triggers Gut Dysbiosis, Neuroinflammation, Gut-Brain Axis Dysfunction, and Vulnerability for Dementia," *CNS & Neurological Disorders - Drug Targets* 14(1) (February 2015): 110-31 (22). Available at http://www.ingentaconnect.com/content/ben/cnsnddt/2014/00000014/00000001/art00018.

154 Kharrazian, Datis. *Why Isn't My Brain Working?*, 126-31.

155 Perlmutter, David E. *Grain Brain*, 21-177.

156 Hollon, Justin et al. "Effect of gliadin on permeability of intestinal biopsy explants from celiac disease patients and patients with non-celiac gluten sensitivity," *Nutrients* 7.3 (2015): 1565-576.

157 Hollon, Justin et al. "Effect of gliadin on permeability of intestinal biopsy explants from celiac disease patients and patients with non-celiac gluten sensitivity." *Nutrients* 7.3 (2015): 1565-576.

158 Severance, Emily G et al. "Subunit and whole molecule specificity of the anti-bovine casein immune response in recent onset psychosis and schizophrenia." Schizophrenia Research 118.1 (2010): 240-47.

159 Kharrazian, Datis. *Why In't My Brain Working?*, 151-152.

160 Brogan, K., MD. "Two Foods That May Sabotage Your Brain." Kelly Brogan MD, (2014, May). Retrieved September 10, 2017, from http://kellybroganmd.com/two-foods-may-sabotage-brain/.

161 Kharrazian, Datis,. *Why Isn't My Brain Working?*, 126, 151-52.

162 Brogan, K., MD. "Two Foods That May Sabotage Your Brain." Kelly Brogan MD, (2014, May). Retrieved September 10, 2017, from http://kellybroganmd.com/two-foods-may-sabotage-brain/.

163 Huebner, FR et al. "Demonstration of high opioid-like activity in isolated peptides from wheat gluten hydrolysates" *Peptides* 5.6 (1984): 1139-147.

[164] Bansal, Vishal et al. "Traumatic brain injury and intestinal dysfunction: uncovering the neuro-enteric axis," *Journal of Neurotrauma* 26.8 (2009): 1353-359.

[165] Forsyth, Christopher B et al. "Increased intestinal permeability correlates with sigmoid mucosa alpha-synuclein staining and endotoxin exposure markers in early Parkinson's disease," *PlOS ONE* 6.12 (2011): e28032.

[166] Hamada, Kazuma et al. "Zonula Occludens-1 alterations and enhanced intestinal permeability in methotrexate-treated rats," *Cancer Chemotherapy and Pharmacology* 66.6 (2010): 1031-038.

[167] Bjarnason, Ingvar et al. "Intestinal permeability and inflammation in rheumatoid arthritis: effects of non-steroidal anti-inflammatory drugs," *The Lancet* 324.8413 (1984): 1171-174.

[168] Fasano, Alessio. "Zonulin and Its Regulation of Intestinal Barrier function: The Biological Door to Inflammation, Autoimmunity, and Cancer," *Physiological Reviews* 91.1 (2011): 151-175.

[169] Hadjivassiliou, Marios, Clare A Williamson, and Nicola Woodroofe. "The immunology of gluten sensitivity: beyond the gut." *Trends in Immunology* 25.11 (2004): 578-82.

[170] Lundin, Knut EA and Armin Alaedini. "Non-celiac gluten sensitivity," *Gastrointestinal Endoscopy Clinics of North America* 22.4 (2012): 723-34.

[171] Bernard, H et al. "Molecular basis of IgE cross-reactivity between human β-casein and bovine β-casein, a major allergen of milk." *Molecular Immunology* 37.3 (2000): 161-167.

[172] Gropper, Sareen S, Jack L Smith, and James L Groff. "Advanced nutrition and human metabolism." *Wadsworth: Wadsworth Cengage Learning* (2009).

[173] Wahls, Terry L. *The Wahls Protocol*, 323-25.

[174] Wahls, Terry L. *The Wahls Protocol*, 323-25.

[175] Wahls, Terry L. *The Wahls Protocol,* 323-25.

[176] Wahls, Terry L. *The Wahls Protocol,* 323-25.

[177] O'Bryan, Tom. *The Autoimmune Fix,* 211-87.

[178] Kharrazian, Datis. *Why Isn't My Brain Working?*, 36-38, 42-43, 101-102, 175.

[179] Perlmutter, David E. *Grain Brain,* 51, 53, 61-62.

[180] Brogan, K., MD. "Two Foods That May Sabotage Your Brain." Kelly Brogan MD, (2014, May). Retrieved September 10, 2017, from http://kellybroganmd.com/two-foods-may-sabotage-brain/.

[181] Perlmutter, David E. *Grain Brain,* 126, 151-52.

[182] Kharrazian, Datis, *Why Isn't My Brain Working?*, 149.

[183] Watts, David L. "Nutrient interrelationships: minerals, vitamins, endocrines," *Journal of Orthomolecular Medicine* 5.1 (1990): 11-19.

[184] O'Dell, Boyd L. "Mineral interactions relevant to nutrient requirements," *The Journal of Nutrition* 119.12 Suppl (1989): 1832-838.

[185] O'Shaughnessy, Thomas J, Hsingch J Lin, and Wu Ma. "Functional synapse formation among rat cortical neurons grown on three-dimensional collagen gels," *Neuroscience Letters* 340.3 (2003): 169-72.

[186] Mahmood A. Aljumaily "The effect of concentrated bone broth as a dietary supplementation on bone healing in rabbits," *Annals of the College of Medicine Mosul* 37 (December 2011): 42-47.

[187] Ihanamäki, Tapio, Lauri J Pelliniemi, and Eero Vuorio. "Collagens and collagen-related matrix components in the human and mouse eye," *Progress in Retinal and Eye Research* 23.4 (2004): 403-34.

[188] Reynolds, Edward. "Vitamin B12, folic acid, and the nervous system," *The Lancet Neurology* 5.11 (2006): 949-60.

[189] Petrucci, Kellyann. *Dr. Kellyann's Bone Broth Diet: Lose Up to 15 Pounds, 4 Inches—and Your Wrinkles!—in Just 21 Days*, (New York: Rodale Press, Inc., 2015), 84.

[191] Wahls, Terry L. *The Wahls Protocol*, 111-12.

[192] Reynolds, Edward. "Vitamin B12, folic acid, and the nervous system," *The Lancet Neurology* 5.11 (2006): 949-60.

[193] Tang, G. "Bioconversion of dietary provitamin A carotenoids to vitamin A in humans," *Am. J of Clin. Nutrition* 91(suppl) (2010): 1468S-1473S. doi:10.3945/ajcn.2010.28674G.

[194] Xiang, Mengqing et al. "Brn-3b: a POU domain gene expressed in a subset of retinal ganglion cells." *Neuron* 11.4 (1993): 689-701.

[195] Bender, David A. *Introduction to Nutrition and Metabolism*, 317-23.

[196] Saari, John C et al. "Cellular retinaldehyde-binding protein is expressed by oligodendrocytes in optic nerve and brain," *Glia* 21.3 (1997): 259-68.

[197] Kennes, B et al. "Effect of vitamin C supplements on cell-mediated immunity in old people," *Gerontology* 29.5 (1983): 305-10.

[198] Anderson, R et al. "The effects of increasing weekly doses of ascorbate on certain cellular and humoral immune functions in normal volunteers," *The American Journal of Clinical Nutrition* 33.1 (1980): 71-76.

[199] Bender, David A. *Introduction to Nutrition and Metabolism*, 366-71.

[200] Ferland, Guylaine. "Vitamin K and the nervous system: an overview of its actions," *Advances in Nutrition: An International Review Journal* 3.2 (2012): 204-212.

[201] Fan, Ying et al. "A preliminary study on bioactivity of orange and tangerine peel extracts against aphis and mites," *Zhongguo Zhong yao za zhi= Zhongguo zhongyao zazhi= China Journal of Chinese Materia Medica* 20.7 (1995): 397-8, 446.

[202] Wahls, Terry L. *The Wahls Protocol*, 116-22.

[203] Trinh, K., et al. "Induction of the Phase II Detoxification Pathway Suppresses Neuron Loss in Drosophila Models of Parkinson's Disease," *J of Neuroscience* 28 (2) (January 9, 2008) 465-472. doi: 10.1523/JNEUROSCI.4778-07.2008 Available at http://www.jneurosci.org/content/28/2/465.short.

[204] Lucas, Sian-Marie, Nancy J Rothwell, and Rosemary M Gibson. "The role of inflammation in CNS injury and disease," *British Journal of Pharmacology* 147.S1 (2006): S232-S240.

[205] O'Dwyer, Sarah T et al. "A single dose of endotoxin increases intestinal permeability in healthy humans," *Archives of Surgery* 123.12 (1988): 1459-464.

[206] Mann, Douglas L. "Stress activated cytokines and the heart," *Cytokine & Growth Factor Reviews* 7.4 (1996): 341-54.

[207] Schmitt, W. "Issue 31 – Cytokines & Liver." Dr. Wally Schmitt, (2015, July 18). Retrieved September 10, 2017, from Issue 31 – Cytokines & Liver .

[208] "The Liver and Detoxification"· Retrieved October 01, 2017, from https://www.liverdoctor.com/liver/the-liver-and-detoxification/.

[209] Wang, Rui. "Physiological implications of hydrogen sulfide: a whiff exploration that blossomed," *Physiological Reviews* 92.2 (2012): 791-896.

[210] Cipolla, Marilyn J. "Anatomy and ultrastructure" *The Cerebral Circulation* (2009).

[211] Dolan, RJ et al. "Regional cerebral blood flow abnormalities in depressed patients with cognitive impairment," *Journal of Neurology, Neurosurgery & Psychiatry* 55.9 (1992): 768-73.

[212] Dolan, RJ et al. "Regional cerebral blood flow abnormalities in depressed patients with cognitive impairment, *Journal of Neurology, Neurosurgery & Psychiatry* 55.9 (1992): 768-73.

[213] Kerns, Michelle L., et al. "Reprogramming of keratin biosynthesis by sulforaphane restores skin integrity in epidermolysis bullosa simplex," *PNAS* 2007 104 (36) 14460-14465; published ahead of print August 27, 2007, doi:10.1073/pnas.0706486104.

[214] Wahls, Terry L. *The Wahls Protocol*, 117.

[215] Guerrero-Beltrán, Carlos Enrique et al. "Protective effect of sulforaphane against oxidative stress: recent advances," *Experimental and Toxicologic Pathology* 64.5 (2012): 503-508.

[216] Wahls, Terry L. *The Wahls Protocol*, 121.

[217] Bianchini, Franca and Harri Vainio. "Allium vegetables and organosulfur compounds: Do they help prevent cancer?" *Environmental Health Perspectives* 109.9 (2001): 893.

[218] Takahashi, Mizuho and Takayuki Shibamoto. "Chemical compositions and antioxidant/anti-inflammatory activities of steam distillate from freeze-dried onion (Allium cepa L.) sprout," *Journal of Agricultural and Food Chemistry* 56.22 (2008): 10462-10467.

[219] Borek, Carmia. "Garlic reduces dementia and heart-disease risk," *The Journal of Nutrition* 136.3 (2006): 810S-812S.

[220] Wahls, Terry L. *The Wahls Protocol*, 119.

[221] Wahls, Terry L. *The Wahls Protocol*, 117, 119, 287.

[222] Wahls, Terry L. *The Wahls Protocol*, 287.

[223] Lull, Cristina, Harry J Wichers, and Huub FJ Savelkoul. "Antiinflammatory and immunomodulating properties of fungal metabolites," *Mediators of*

Inflammation 2005.2 (2005): 63-80.

²²⁴ Akramiene, Dalia et al. "Effects of beta-glucans on the immune system," *Medicina (Kaunas, Lithuania)* 43.8 (2006): 597-606.

²²⁵ Wahls, Terry L. *The Wahls Protocol*, 120.

²²⁶ Wahls, Terry L. *The Wahls Protocol*, 113-14.

²²⁷ Wahls, Terry L. *The Wahls Protocol*, 114.

²²⁸ Wahls, Terry L. *The Wahls Protocol*, 114.

²²⁹ Wahls, Terry L. *The Wahls Protocol*, 142.

²³⁰ Ames, Bruce N, Mark K Shigenaga, and Tory M Hagen. "Oxidants, antioxidants, and the degenerative diseases of aging," *Proceedings of the National Academy of Sciences* 90.17 (1993): 7915-922.

²³¹ Ames, Bruce N, Mark K Shigenaga, and Tory M Hagen. "Oxidants, antioxidants, and the degenerative diseases of aging" 7915-922.

²³² Ames, Bruce N, Mark K Shigenaga, and Tory M Hagen. "Oxidants, antioxidants, and the degenerative diseases of aging" 7915-922.

²³³ Ames, Bruce N, Mark K Shigenaga, and Tory M Hagen. "Oxidants, antioxidants, and the degenerative diseases of aging" 7915-922.

²³⁴ Slemmer, Jennifer E et al. "Antioxidants and free radical scavengers for the treatment of stroke, traumatic brain injury and aging," *Current Medicinal Chemistry* 15.4 (2008): 404-14.

²³⁵ Giunta, Brian et al. "The immunology of traumatic brain injury: a prime target for Alzheimer's disease prevention," *Journal of Neuroinflammation* 9.1 (2012): 185.

236 Shao, ChangXing et al. "Oxidative stress in head trauma in aging," *Free Radical Biology and Medicine* 41.1 (2006): 77-85.

237 Watzl, Bernhard. "Anti-inflammatory effects of plant-based foods and of their constituents," *International Journal for Vitamin and Nutrition Research* 78.6 (2008): 293-298.

238 Youdim, Kuresh A. and James A. Joseph. "A possible emerging role of phytochemicals in improving age-related neurological dysfunctions: a multiplicity of effects," *Free Radical Biology and Medicine* 30.6 (2001): 583-94.

239 Webb, Andrew J et al. "Acute blood pressure lowering, vasoprotective, and antiplatelet properties of dietary nitrate via bioconversion to nitrite," *Hypertension* 51.3 (2008): 784-90.

240 The Institute of Functional Medicine "Phytonutrient-Spectrum-Comprehensive-Guide" (2014). Retrieved on 30 Apr. 2016 http://www.thehealthedgepodcast.com/wp-content/uploads/2015/07/Phytonutrient-Spectrum-Comprehensive-Guide.pdf.

241 Wahls, Terry L. *The Wahls Protocol*, 372.

242 Wahls, Terry L. *The Wahls Protocol*, 373.

243 Wahls, Terry L. *The Wahls Protocol*, 374.

244 Wahls, Terry L. *The Wahls Protocol*, 374.

245 Wahls, Terry L. *The Wahls Protocol*, 116.

246 Münch, Gerald et al. "Advanced glycation endproducts and their pathogenic roles in neurological disorders," *Amino Acids* 42.4 (2012): 1221-236.

247 Emanuele, Enzo et al. "Circulating levels of soluble receptor for advanced glycation end products in Alzheimer disease and vascular dementia," *Archives of Neurology* 62.11 (2005): 1734-736.

²⁴⁸ Coker, Laura H. and Lynne E. Wagenknecht. "Advanced glycation end products, diabetes, and the brain," *Neurology* 77.14 (2011): 1326-327.

²⁴⁹ Curtis, TM et al. "Müller glial dysfunction during diabetic retinopathy in rats is linked to accumulation of advanced glycation end-products and advanced lipoxidation end-products," *Diabetologia* 54.3 (2011): 690-98.

²⁵⁰ Batty, G David et al. "IQ in early adulthood and mortality by middle age: cohort study of 1 million Swedish men," *Epidemiology* 20.1 (2009): 100-09.

²⁵¹ Scheele, Camilla et al. "Altered regulation of the PINK1 locus: a link between Type 2 diabetes and neurodegeneration?" *The FASEB Journal* 21.13 (2007): 3653-665.

²⁵² Suzanne, M. and Jack R Wands. "Alzheimer's disease is Type 3 diabetes—evidence reviewed." *Journal of Diabetes Science and Technology* 2.6 (2008): 1101-113.

²⁵³ Kharrazian, Datis. *Why Isn't My Brain Working?*, 71.

²⁵⁴ Permlutter, David E. *Grain Brain*, 27-31.

²⁵⁵ Kharrazian, Datis. *Why Isn't My Brain Working?*, 59-71.

²⁵⁶ Suh, Sang Won et al. "Hypoglycemic neuronal death is triggered by glucose reperfusion and activation of neuronal NADPH oxidase," *The Journal of Clinical Investigation* 117.4 (2007): 910-18.

²⁵⁷ Kharrazian, Datis. *Why Isn't My Brain Working?*, 63-64.

²⁵⁸ Kikuchi, Seiji et al. "Glycation—a sweet tempter for neuronal death., *Brain Research Reviews* 41.2 (2003): 306-23.

²⁵⁹ Kikuchi, Seiji et al. "Glycation—a sweet tempter for neuronal death" 306-323.

[260] Perlmutter, David E. *Grain Brain*, 113-14.

[261] Juvenile Diabetes Research Foundation Continuous Glucose Monitoring Study Group. "Variation of interstitial glucose measurements assessed by continuous glucose monitors in healthy, nondiabetic individuals," *Diabetes Care* 33.6 (2010): 1297-299.

[262] Nakayama, Andrea. Transcript of Sweet Tooth Bitter Truth: Sugar in Your Body and Brain (Replenish PDX), p. 19. (obtained by the author as part of the Sweet Tooth Bitter Truth: Sugar in Your Body and Brain course offered by Replenish PDX, now known as Functional Nutrition Alliance).

[263] Munck, Allan, and Seymour B Koritz. "Studies on the mode of action of glucocorticoids in rats I. Early effects of cortisol on blood glucose and on glucose entry into muscle, liver and adiposèttissue," *Biochimica et Biophysica Acta* 57.1 (1962): 310-17.

[264] Weitzman, Elliot D et al. "Twenty-four hour pattern of the episodic secretion of cortisol in normal subjects," *The Journal of Clinical Endocrinology & Metabolism* 33.1 (1971): 14-22.

[265] Rizza, Robert A, Lawrence J Mandarino, and John E Gerich. "Cortisol-Induced Insulin Resistance in Man: Impaired Suppression of Glucose Production and Stimulation of Glucose Utilization due to a Postreceptor Defect of Insulin Action," *The Journal of Clinical Endocrinology & Metabolism* 54.1 (1982): 131-38.

[266] Bolton, Robin P, Kenneth W Heaton, and Lennard F Burroughs. "The role of dietary fiber in satiety, glucose, and insulin: studies with fruit and fruit juice," *The American Journal of Clinical Nutrition* 34.2 (1981): 211-17.

[267] The NIH HMP Working Group, "The NIH Human Microbiome Project" Genome Res. 19 (2009): 2317-2323. Also available online at http://www.genome.org/cgi/doi/10.1101/gr.096651.109.

[268] Wikipedia, "Human Microbiome Project" availabe at https://en.wikipedia.org/wiki/Human_Microbiome_Project.

[269] Arthur, Benjamin and Rob Stein. "Exploring The Invisible Universe That Lives On Us — And In Us," National Public Radio (November 4, 2013). Retrieved on September 29, 2017 from http://www.npr.org/sections/health-shots/2013/11/01/242361826/exploring-the-invisible-universe-that-lives-on-us-and-in-us. Part of an NPR special series called The Human Microbiome: Guts and Glory (http://www.npr.org/series/218987212/microbiome).

[270] Pflughoeft, Kathryn J. and James Versalovic. "Human microbiome in health and disease," *Annual Review of Pathology: Mechanisms of Disease* 7 (2012): 99-122.

[271] Gerritsen, Jacoline et al. "Intestinal microbiota in human health and disease: the impact of probiotics." *Genes & Nutrition* 6.3 (2011): 209-40.

[272] Wahls, Terry. *The Wahls Protocol*, 90.

[273] Wahls, Terry. *The Wahls Protocol*, 90.

[274] McFall-Ngai, M., et al. "Animals in a bacterial world, a new imperative for the life sciences," *PNAS* 110 (9) (2013): 3229-236; published ahead of print February 7, 2013, doi:10.1073/pnas.1218525110.

[275] Velasquez-Manoff, M. "Fruits and Vegetables Are Trying to Kill You," *Nautilus*, (2014, July 17). doi:http://nautil.us/issue/15/turbulence/fruits-and-vegetables-are-trying-to-kill-you.

[276] Mattson, Mark P. and Aiwu Cheng. "Neurohormetic phytochemicals: Low-dose toxins that induce adaptive neuronal stress responses," *Trends in Neurosciences* 29.11 (2006): 632-39.

[277] Mattson, Mark P. and Aiwu Cheng. "Neurohormetic phytochemicals" 632-39.

[278] Ogden, Cynthia L., et al. "Prevalence of overweight and obesity in the United States, 1999-2004," *JAMA* 295.13 (2006): 1549-555.

[279] Ng, Marie, et al. "Global, regional, and national prevalence of overweight and obesity in children and adults during 1980–2013: A Systematic Analysis for the Global Burden of Disease Study 2013," *The Lancet* 384.9945 (2014): 766-81.

[280] Gasior, Maciej, Michael A Rogawski, and Adam L Hartman. "Neuroprotective and disease-modifying effects of the ketogenic diet," *Behavioural Pharmacology* 17.5-6 (2006): 431.

[281] Maalouf, Marwan, Jong M Rho, and Mark P Mattson. "The neuroprotective properties of calorie restriction, the ketogenic diet, and ketone bodies." *Brain Research Reviews* 59.2 (2009): 293-315.

[282] Neuringer, Martha and William E. Connor. "N-3 Fatty Acids in the Brain and Retina: Evidence for Their Essentiality," *Nutrition Reviews* 44.9 (2009): 285-94.

[283] Haag, Marianne. "Essential fatty acids and the brain." *Canadian Journal of Psychiatry. Revue Cnadienne de Psychiatrie* 48.3 (2003): 195-203.

[284] Wainwright, Patricia E. "Dietary essential fatty acids and brain function: a developmental perspective on mechanisms." *Proceedings of the Nutrition Society* 61.01 (2002): 61-69.

[285] Innis, Sheila M. "Dietary (n-3) fatty acids and brain development," *The Journal of Nutrition* 137.4 (2007): 855-59.

[286] Center for Disease Control and Prevention. "CDC Prevention Guidelines." Public Health Service, (1989, October 01). Retrieved September 11, 2017, from https://wonder.cdc.gov/wonder/prevguid/p0000109/p0000109.asp#head021000000000000.

[287] Cunnane, S. C., & Crawford, M. A. "Energetic and nutritional constraints on infant brain development: Implications for brain expansion during human evolution." *J of Human Evolution,* 77 (2014): 88-98. doi:10.1016/j.jhevol.2014.05.001

[288] Perlmutter, David E. *Grain Brain.* 185-186.

[289] Barañano K.W. and Hartman, A.L. "The ketogenic diet: uses in epilepsy and other neurologic illnesses," *Curr Treat Options Neurol.* 10(6)(2008 Nov): 410-19.

[290] Farooqui, A., et al. "Modulation of inflammation in brain: a matter of fat," *J of Neurochemistry*, 101(3) (2006): 577-99. doi:10.1111/j.1471-4159.2006.04371.x.

[291] Chen, C. "Lipids: COX-2s new role in inflammation," *Nature Chemical Biology*, 6(6) (2010): 401-02. doi:10.1038/nchembio.375.

[292] So, J. K. (1980). "Human Biological Adaptation to Arctic and Subarctic Zones," *Annual Review of Anthropology*, 9(1), 63-82. doi:10.1146/annurev.an.09.100180.000431.

[293] Sejian, V., Maurya, V. P., and Naqvi, S. M. "Adaptive capability as indicated by endocrine and biochemical responses of Malpura ewes subjected to combined stresses (thermal and nutritional) in a semi-arid tropical environment." *Intl J of Biometeorology*, 54(6) (2010): 653-61. doi:10.1007/s00484-010-0341-1

[294] Reger, Mark A et al. "Effects of β-hydroxybutyrate on cognition in memory-impaired adults," *Neurobiology of Aging* 25.3 (2004): 311-14.

[295] Gasior, Maciej, Michael A Rogawski, and Adam L Hartman. "Neuroprotective and disease-modifying effects of the ketogenic diet," *Behavioural Pharmacology* 17.5-6 (2006): 431.

[296] Morris, Martha Clare et al. "Dietary fats and the risk of incident Alzheimer disease," *Archives of Neurology* 60.2 (2003): 194-200.

[297] Vanitallie, TB et al. "Treatment of Parkinson disease with diet-induced hyperketonemia: a feasibility study," *Neurology* 64.4 (2005): 728-30.

[298] Prins, ML, LS Fujima, and DA Hovda. "Age-dependent reduction of cortical contusion volume by ketones after traumatic brain injury," *Journal of Neuroscience Research* 82.3 (2005): 413-20.

[299] Yamada, Kelvin A., Nicholas Rensing, and Liu Lin Thio. "Ketogenic diet reduces hypoglycemia-induced neuronal death in young rats," *Neuroscience Letters* 385.3 (2005): 210-14.

[300] Swink, Traci D., EP Vining, and John M. Freeman. "The Ketogenic Diet: 1997," *Advances in Pediatrics* 44 (1996): 297-329.

[301] Stafstrom, C.E. and Rho, J.M. "The Ketogenic Diet as a Treatment for Diverse Neurological Disorders," *Frontiers in Pharmaology* 3 (2012): 59.

[302] BreakNutrition· "What is the keto flu or low carb flu and what to do about it?" (September 19, 2017). Retrieved September 30, 2017, from http://breaknutrition.com/keto-flu/.

[303] Wilson, J. M. and Lowery, R. *The Ketogenic Bible: The Authoritative Guide to Ketosis* (Las Vegas: Victory Belt Publishing, 2017).

[304] Kalamian, M. *Keto for Cancer: Ketogenic Metabolic Therapy as a Targeted Nutritional Strategy* (White River Junction, VT: Chelsea Green Publishing, 2017), 27.

[305] de Souza, Russell J et al. "Intake of saturated and trans unsaturated fatty acids and risk of all cause mortality, cardiovascular disease, and Type 2 diabetes: systematic review and meta-analysis of observational studies," *BMJ* 351 (2015): h3978.

[306] Chowdhury, Rajiv et al. "Association of dietary, circulating, and supplement fatty acids with coronary risk: a systematic review and meta-analysis." *Annals of Internal Medicine* 160.6 (2014): 398-406.

[307] Schwab, Ursula et al. "Effect of the amount and type of dietary fat on cardiometabolic risk factors and risk of developing Type-2 diabetes, cardiovascular disease, and cancer: a systematic review," *Food & Nutrition Research* 58 (2014).

[308] Walsh, B. "Ending the War on Fat." *Time Magazine,* 183(24) (2014, June 23).

[309] Okie, Susan. "New York to trans fats: you're out!" *New England Journal of Medicine* 356.20 (2007): 2017-021.

[310] Mozaffarian, Dariush et al. "Trans fatty acids and cardiovascular disease," *New England Journal of Medicine* 354.15 (2006): 1601-613.

[311] Kummerow, Fred A. "The negative effects of hydrogenated trans fats and what to do about them." *Atherosclerosis* 205.2 (2009): 458-65.

[312] Przybylski, Roman, et al. "Canola oil." Chapter 2 of *Bailey's Industrial Oil & Fat Products: Volume 2: Edible oil and fat products: edible oils*, ed. Fereidoon Shahidi (Hoboken, NJ: John Wiley & Sons, 2005), 61-121. DOI: 10.1002/047167849X.bio004.

[313] Finkelstein, Israel and Neil Asher Silberman. *David and Solomon: In Search of the Bible's Sacred Kings and the Roots of the Western Tradition* (New York: Free Press, 2006), 131, 317.

[314] Covas, María-Isabel et al. "Minor components of olive oil: evidence to date of health benefits in humans," *Nutrition Reviews* 64. suppl 4 (2006): S20-S30.

[315] Fulgoni, V. L., Dreher, M., and Davenport, A. J. "Avocado consumption is associated with better diet quality and nutrient intake, and lower metabolic syndrome risk in US adults: results from the National Health and Nutrition Examination Survey (NHANES) 2001–2008," *Nutrition Journal* 12(1) (2013). doi:10.1186/1475-2891-12-1

[316] Ogbolu, DO et al. "In vitro antimicrobial properties of coconut oil on Candida species in Ibadan, Nigeria," *Journal of Medicinal Food* 10.2 (2007): 384-387.

[317] Esterbauer, Hermann. "Cytotoxicity and genotoxicity of lipid-oxidation products," *The American Journal of Clinical Nutrition* 57.5 (1993): 779S-785S.

[318] Alexander, JC. "Chemical and biological properties related to toxicity of heated fats," *Journal of Toxicology and Environmental Health, Part A Current*

Issues 7.1 (1981): 125-38.

319 Staprans, Ilona et al. "Oxidized lipids in the diet are a source of oxidized lipid in chylomicrons of human serum." *Arteriosclerosis, Thrombosis, and Vascular Biology* 14.12 (1994): 1900-905.

320 Jaarin, Kamsiah and Yusof Kamisah. "Repeatedly Heated Vegetable Oils and Lipid Peroxidation." *Lipid Peroxidation*, 2012. doi:10.5772/46076.

321 Addis, PB. "Occurrence of lipid oxidation products in foods." *Food and Chemical Toxicology* 24.10 (1986): 1021-030.

322 Przybylski, Roman et al. "Canola oil," *Bailey's Industrial Oil and Fat Products* (2005).

323 Taubes, Gary. *Good calories, bad calories: Fats, carbs, and the controversial science of diet and health.* (New York: Anchor Books, 2008).

324 Johnstone, Alexandra M et al. "Effects of a high-protein ketogenic diet on hunger, appetite, and weight loss in obese men feeding ad libitum," *The American Journal of Clinical Nutrition* 87.1 (2008): 44-55.

325 Sondike, Stephen B, Nancy Copperman, and Marc S Jacobson. "Effects of a low-carbohydrate diet on weight loss and cardiovascular risk factor in overweight adolescents," *The Journal of Pediatrics* 142.3 (2003): 253-58.

326 Cholesterol Numbers video on Mayo Clinic website. Retrieved September 23, 2017 from http://www.mayoclinic.org/cholesterol-numbers-video/vid-20078243.

327 Gasior, Maciej, Michael A. Rogawski, and Adam L. Hartman. "Neuroprotective and disease-modifying effects of the ketogenic diet," *Behavioural Pharmacology* 17.5-6 (2006): 431.

328 Elias, Ellen, et al. "Clinical effects of cholesterol supplementation in six patients with the Smith-Lemli-Opitz syndrome (SLOS)," *American Journal of*

Medical Genetics (1997): 305-10.

[329] Elias, Ellen, et al. "Clinical effects of cholesterol supplementation in six patients with the Smith-Lemli-Opitz syndrome (SLOS)" 305-10.

[330] Elias, Ellen, et al. "Clinical effects of cholesterol supplementation in six patients with the Smith-Lemli-Opitz syndrome (SLOS)" 305-10.

[331] Davison, Karen M., and Bonnie J. Kaplan. "Lipophilic Statin Use and Suicidal Ideation in a Sample of Adults With Mood Disorders," *Crisis* 35.4 (2014): 278-82.

[332] Hanukoglu, Israel. "Steroidogenic enzymes: Structure, function, and role in regulation of steroid hormone biosynthesis," *The Journal of Steroid Biochemistry and Molecular Biology* (1992): 779-804.

[333] Perlmutter, David E. *Grain Brain*, 93-98.

[334] Perlmutter, David. E. *Grain Brain*, 91.

[335] Pfrieger, Frank. "Role of cholesterol in synapse formation and function," *Biochimica et Biophysica Acta (BBA) - Biomembranes* (2003): 271-80.

[336] Pfrieger, Frank. "Role of cholesterol in synapse formation and function" 271-80.

[337] Baron, Stephen and Phillip Hylemon. "Biotransformation of Bile Acids, Cholesterol, and Steroid Hormones." *Gastrointestinal Microbiology* (1997): 470-510.

[338] Perlmutter, David E. *Grain Brain*, 91-93.

[339] Sachinidis, A., R. Kettenhofen, S. Seewald, I. Gouni-Berthold, U. Schmitz, C. Seul, Y. Ko, and H. Vetter "Evidence That Lipoproteins Are Carriers of Bioactive Factors." *Arteriosclerosis, Thrombosis, and Vascular Biology* (1999): 2412-421.

340 Perlmutter, David E. *Grain Brain,* 92, 100-102.

341 Perlmutter, David E. *Grain Brain,* 91.

342 Koenig, W. et al. "C-reactive protein, a sensitive marker for inflammation, predicts future risk of coronary heart disease in initially healthy middle-aged men," *Journal of Cardiothoracic and Vascular Anesthesia* (1999): 237-42.

343 Koenig, W. et al. "C-reactive protein, a sensitive marker for inflammation, predicts future risk of coronary heart disease in initially healthy middle-aged men" 237-42.

344 Datta, Subinay, Zahidul Iqbal, and K.R. Prasad. "Comparison Between Serum hsCRP and LDL Cholesterol for Search of a Better Predictor for Ischemic Heart Disease," *Indian Journal of Clinical Biochemistry* (2011): 210-13.

345 Datta, Subinay, Zahidul Iqbal, and K.R. Prasad. "Comparison Between Serum hsCRP and LDL Cholesterol for Search of a Better Predictor for Ischemic Heart Disease," *Indian Journal of Clinical Biochemistry* (2011): 210-13.

346 Fernandez, Maria. "Rethinking dietary cholesterol." *Current Opinion in Clinical Nutrition and Metabolic Care* (2012): 117-21.

347 Perlmutter, David E. *Grain Brain,* 98-100.

348 Perlmutter, David E. *Grain Brain,* 93-100.

349 Perlmutter, David E. *Grain Brain,* 93-100.

350 Kannappan, Ramaswamy et al. "Neuroprotection by spice-derived nutraceuticals: you are what you eat!." *Molecular Neurobiology* 44.2 (2011): 142-59.

351 Singletary, Keith. "Black pepper: overview of health benefits," *Nutrition Today* 45.1 (2010): 43-47.

352 Elkaim, Y. "The Truth About How Much Water You Should Really Drink."

(September 13, 2013). Retrieved September 30, 2017, from https://health. usnews.com/health-news/blogs/eat-run/2013/09/13/the-truth-about-how-much-water-you-should-really-drink

353 Prentice, A. (2005). "Macronutrients as sources of food energy," *Public Health Nutrition*, 8(7a), 932-39. doi:10.1079/PHN2005779

354 Wahls, Terry L. *The Wahls Protocol*, 197.

355 Pfrieger, Frank W. "Role of cholesterol in synapse formation and function," *Biochimica et Biophysica Acta (BBA)-Biomembranes* 1610.2 (2003): 271-80.

356 Kharrazian, Datis. *Why Isn't My Brain Working?*, 28-30.

357 Kharrazian, Datis. *Why Isn't My Brain Working?*, 22-26, 30-31.

358 Wurtman, Richard J et al. "Use of phosphatide precursors to promote synaptogenesis," *Annual Review of Nutrition* 29 (2009): 59-87.

359 Wurtman, Richard J. "Enhancing synaptogenesis in diseases characterized by deficiencies in brain synapses," *Frontiers in Psychiatry* 1 (2010).

360 Blusztajn, Jan K, and Richard J Wurtman. "Choline biosynthesis by a preparation enriched in synaptosomes from rat brain." *Nature* 290.5805 (1981): 417-18.

361 Wurtman, Richard J. "A nutrient combination that can affect synapse formation, *Nutrients* 6.4 (2014): 1701-710.

362 Wurtman, Richard J. et al. "Nutritional modifiers of aging brain function: use of uridine and other phosphatide precursors to increase formation of brain synapses," *Nutrition Reviews* 68. suppl 2 (2010): S88-S101.

363 Wurtman, Richard J. et al. "Synaptic proteins and phospholipids are increased in gerbil brain by administering uridine plus docosahexaenoic acid orally," *Brain Research* 1088.1 (2006): 83-92.

[364] Wurtman, Richard J. et al. "Synaptic proteins and phospholipids are increased in gerbil brain by administering uridine plus docosahexaenoic acid orally" 83-92.

[365] Blalock, T. "Citicoline Vs. Choline." Livestrong, (October 11, 2015). Retrieved September 10, 2017, from http://www.livestrong.com/article/478224-citicoline-vs-choline/.

[366] Hasselmo, Michael E. "Neuromodulation and cortical function: modeling the physiological basis of behavior," *Behavioural Brain Research* 67.1 (1995): 1-27.

[367] Hasselmo, Michael E. "Neuromodulation and cortical function: modeling the physiological basis of behavior" 1-27.

[368] Teather, Lisa A, and Richard J Wurtman. "Dietary CDP-choline supplementation prevents memory impairment caused by impoverished environmental conditions in rats," *Learning & Memory* 12.1 (2005): 39-43.

[369] Baskaya, Mustafa K et al. "Neuroprotective effects of citicoline on brain edema and blood-brain barrier breakdown after traumatic brain injury," *Journal of Neurosurgery* 92.3 (2000): 448-52.

[370] EFSA NDA Panel (EFSA Panel on Dietetic Products, Nutrition and Allergies), 2013. "Scientific Opinion on the safety of "citicoline" as a Novel Food ingredient," *EFSA Journal* 11 (10) (2013):3421-22 pp. doi:10.2903/j.efsa.2013.3421

[371] Lewis, Michael, Parviz Ghassemi, and Joseph Hibbeln. "Therapeutic use of omega-3 fatty acids in severe head trauma," *The American Journal of Emergency Medicine* 31.1 (2013): 273. e5-273. e8.

[372] Lewis, Michael D. and Julian Bailes. "Neuroprotection for the warrior: dietary supplementation with omega-3 fatty acids," *Military Medicine* 176.10 (2011): 1120-127.

[373] Hasadsri, L., et al. "Omega-3 Fatty Acids as a Putative Treatment for Traumatic Brain Injury, *Journal of Neurotrauma* 30(11) (2013): 897-906.

doi:10.1089/neu.2012.2672.

[374] Wurtman, Richard J et al. "Synaptic proteins and phospholipids are increased in gerbil brain by administering uridine plus docosahexaenoic acid orally," *Brain Research* 1088.1 (2006): 83-92.

[375] Saydoff-Rolando, Joel, et al. "Oral uridine pro-drug PN401 is neuroprotective in the R6/2 and N171-82Q mouse models of Huntington's disease," *Neurobiology of Disease* 24 (3) (2006): 455-65. doi:10.1016/j.nbd.2006.08.011.

[376] Ratey, John J. *A User's Guide to the Brain: Perception, Attention, and the Four Theatres of the Brain* (New York: Vintage Books, 2001).

[377] Wurtman, Richard J et al. "Synaptic proteins and phospholipids are increased in gerbil brain by administering uridine plus docosahexaenoic acid orally," *Brain Research* 1088.1 (2006): 83-92.

[378] Yu, VY. "The role of dietary nucleotides in neonatal and infant nutrition," *Singapore Medical Journal* 39.4 (1998): 145-50.

[379] Carr, Daniel O, and Santiago Grisolia. "Incorporation of dihydrouridine monophosphate and uridine monophosphate into liver and brain ribonucleic acid," *Journal of Biological Chemistry* 239.1 (1964): 160-66.

[380] Borzelleca, J. F. "A Critical Evaluation of the Available Information on the Toxicity/Safety of Orally Administered Uridine." United States Food & Drug Administration, (2002, June 11). Retrieved September 10, 2017, from https://www.fda.gov/ohrms/dockets/dockets/95s0316/95s-0316-rpt0182-02-tab-01-01-vol134-web.pdf.

[381] Wahls, Terry L. *The Wahls Protocol*, 174.

[382] Williams, Peter. "Nutritional composition of red meat," *Nutrition & Dietetics* 64.s4 (2007): S113-S119.

[383] Wahls, Terry L. *The Wahls Protocol*, 184.

[384] Chilton, Stephanie N, Jeremy P Burton, and Gregor Reid. "Inclusion of fermented foods in food guides around the world," *Nutrients* 7.1 (2015): 390-404.

[385] David, Lawrence A., et al. "Diet rapidly and reproducibly alters the human gut microbiome", *Nature* 505.7484 (2014): 559-63.

[386] David, Lawrence A., et al. "Diet rapidly and reproducibly alters the human gut microbiome" 559-63.

[387] Tascher, J. "Sauerkraut: The Most Misunderstood Health Food." Bottom Line Inc, (2017, February 22). RetrievedSeptember 10, 2017, from https://bottomlineinc.com/life/food/sauerkraut-the-most-misunderstood-health-food

[388] Parvez, S et al. "Probiotics and their fermented food products are beneficial for health," *Journal of Applied Microbiology* 100.6 (2006): 1171-185.

[389] Prohaska, Joseph R. "Functions of trace elements in brain metabolism," *Physiological Reviews* 67.3 (1987): 858-901.

[390] Knudsen, Nils et al. "Comparative study of thyroid function and types of thyroid dysfunction in two areas in Denmark with slightly different iodine status," *European Journal of Endocrinology* 143.4 (2000): 485-91.

[391] Doyle, M. "Iodine: The Forgotten Nutrient." Blueprint Fitness, (2009, December 11). Accessed September 10, 2017, from http://www.blueprintfitness.co.uk/iodine-the-forgotten-nutrient/.

[392] Wahls, Terry L. *The Wahls Protocol*, 170.

[393] Wahls, Terry L. *The Wahls Protocol*, 169.

[394] Skoryna, Stanley C, TM Paul, and Deirdre Waldron Edward. "Studies on inhibition of intestinal absorption of radioactive strontium: I. Prevention of absorption from ligated intestinal segments," *Canadian Medical Association Journal* 91.6 (1964): 285.

[395] Skoryna, Stanley C, et al.. "Studies on inhibition of intestinal absorption of radioactive strontium" 285.

[396] Wahls, Terry L. *The Wahls Protocol,* 171.

[397] Wahls, Terry L. *The Wahls Protocol,* 172.

[398] Wahls, Terry L. *The Wahls Protocol,* 150.

[399] Mozaffarian, D. and Rimm, E. "Fish Intake, Contaminants, and Human Health," *JAMA* 296(15) (2006): 1885-899. doi:10.1001/jama.296.15.1885.

[400] Mozaffarian, D. and Rimm, E. "Fish Intake, Contaminants, and Human Health" 1885-899.

[401] Mozaffarian, D. and Rimm, E. "Fish Intake, Contaminants, and Human Health" 1885-899.

[402] Mozaffarian, D. and Rimm, E. "Fish Intake, Contaminants, and Human Health" 1885-899.

[403] Mozaffarian, D. and Rimm, E. "Fish Intake, Contaminants, and Human Health" 1885-899.

[404] Mozaffarian, D. and Rimm, E. "Fish Intake, Contaminants, and Human Health" 1885-899.

[405] Mozaffarian, D. and Rimm, E. "Fish Intake, Contaminants, and Human Health" 1885-899.

[406] Mozaffarian, D. and Rimm, E. "Fish Intake, Contaminants, and Human Health" 1885-899.

[407] Mozaffarian, D. and Rimm, E. "Fish Intake, Contaminants, and Human Health" 1885-899.

[408] Mozaffarian, D. and Rimm, E. "Fish Intake, Contaminants, and Human

Health" 1885-899.

[409] Fallon, A. "'Local' food labeling misleads consumers, regulator reveals," *The Guardian*, (2011, February 25). Retrieved September 10, 2017, from https://www.theguardian.com/environment/2011/feb/26/local-food-labelling-misleading-consumers.

[410] Center for Food Safety and Applied Nutrition. "Labeling & Nutrition." (n.d.). Retrieved September 10, 2017, from https://www.fda.gov/Food/GuidanceRegulation/GuidanceDocumentsRegulatoryInformation/Labeling-Nutrition/ucm456090.htm.

[411] Center for Food Safety and Applied Nutrition. "Labeling & Nutrition." (n.d.). Retrieved September 10, 2017, from https://www.fda.gov/Food/GuidanceRegulation/GuidanceDocumentsRegulatoryInformation/Labeling-Nutrition/ucm456090.htm.

[412] "Natural" on Food Labeling." Food and Drug Administration (2015). Retrieved on 29 Apr. 2016. http://www.fda.gov/Food/GuidanceRegulation/GuidanceDocumentsRegulatoryInformation/LabelingNutrition/ucm456090.htm.

[413] OrganicAuthority.com. "5 Food Labels That Mean Nothing." *Huffington Post*, (2012, January 12). Retrieved September 10, 2017, from http://www.huffingtonpost.com/organic-authoritycom/5-food-labels-that-mean-n_b_1202681.html.

[414] OrganicAuthority.com. "5 Food Labels That Mean Nothing." *Huffington Post*, (2012, January 12). Retrieved September 10, 2017, from http://www.huffingtonpost.com/organic-authoritycom/5-food-labels-that-mean-n_b_1202681.html.

[415] United States Department of Agriculture. "Meat and Poultry Labeling Terms". (n.d.). Retrieved September 10, 2017, from https://www.fsis.usda.gov/wps/portal/fsis/topics/food-safety-education/get-answers/food-safety-fact-sheets/food-labeling/meat-and-poultry-labeling-terms/!ut/p/a1/jVJt-b4IwEP4t-wDfoEWc0SVkIWxmuokxZhvyZSlwvBigrC0S9-tHWTRq1N-

mmues9z13b54p85CG_JJssISKjJcnl3h984QU.

416 The Humane Society of the United States. "How to Read Meat and Dairy Labels." (n.d.). Retrieved September 10, 2017, from http://www.humanesociety.org/issues/confinement_farm/facts/meat_dairy_labels.html#.Uo_GKc-TOmSo.

417 One Green Planet. "Think You Know 'Free-Range' and 'Cage Free' Chicken? Think Again." (2015, November 13). Retrieved September 10, 2017, from http://www.onegreenplanet.org/animalsandnature/think-you-know-free-range-and-cage-free-chicken-think-again/.

418 Séralini, Gilles-Eric, et al. "Answers to critics: Why there is a long term toxicity due to a Roundup-tolerant genetically modified maize and to a Roundup herbicide," *Food and Chemical Toxicology* 53 (2013): 476-483.

419 Séralini, Gilles-Eric, et al. "Answers to critics" 476-83.

420 Schütte, G. et al. "Herbicide resistance and biodiversity: agronomic and environmental aspects of genetically modified herbicide-resistant plants," *Environmental Sciences Europe* 29:5 (2017). Retrieved September 23, 2017 from https://doi.org/10.1186/s12302-016-0100-y.

421 Schütte, G. et al. "Herbicide resistance and biodiversity."

422 University of California, San Diego. "How Does Bt Work." Retrieved September 10, 2017, from http://www.bt.ucsd.edu/how_bt_work.html (This website is created and maintained by the Aroian lab at University of California San Diego, which studies Bt (*bacillus thuringiensis*)).

423 Mesnage, R et al. "Cytotoxicity on human cells of Cry1Ab and Cry1Ac Bt insecticidal toxins alone or with a glyphosate-based herbicide," *Journal of Applied Toxicology* 33.7 (2013): 695-99.

424 Johnson, D., and O'Connor, S. "These Charts Show Every Genetically Modified Food People Already Eat in the U.S." *Time Magazine,* (2015, April 30). Retrieved September 10, 2017, from http://time.com/3840073/gmo-

food-charts/.

425 Fernandez-Cornejo, Jorge, Seth Wechsler, Mike Livingston, Lorraine Mitchell. "Genetically Engineered Crops in the United States." SSRN Electronic Journal (2014).

426 Aldai, Noelia et al. "Length of concentrate finishing affects the fatty acid composition of grass-fed and genetically lean beef: an emphasis on trans-18: 1 and conjugated linoleic acid profiles," *Animal: An International Journal of Animal Bioscience* 5.10 (2011): 1643.

427 Takeuchi, Masayoshi, and Sho-ichi Yamagishi. "Possible involvement of advanced glycation end-products (AGEs) in the pathogenesis of Alzheimer's disease," *Current Pharmaceutical Design* 14.10 (2008): 973-978.

428 O'Keefe, Sean et al. "Levels of Trans Geometrical Isomers of Essential Fatty Acids in Some UnhydrogenatedU.S. Vegetable Oils," *Journal of Food Lipids* 1.3 (1994): 165-176.

429 Rackis, J. J., M.R. Gumbmann, and I.E. Liener. "The USDA trypsin inhibitor study. I. Background, objectives, and procedural details," *Qualitas Plantarum Plant Foods for Human Nutrition* 35(3) (1985): 213-42. doi:10.1007/bf01092196.

430 Lewis, Michael, Parviz Ghassemi, and Joseph Hibbeln. "Therapeutic use of omega-3 fatty acids in severe head trauma," *The American Journal of Emergency Medicine* 31.1 (2013): 273. e5-273. e8.

431 Schoenfeld, Laura. "The Use of Blenderized Tube Feeding in Pediatric Patients: Evidence and Guidelines for Dietetic Practice" (Chapel Hill, North Carolina)." 5 Dec. 2013.

432 Escuro, Arlene A. "Blenderized tube feeding: suggested guidelines to clinicians," *Practical Gastroenterology* (2014).

433 Schoenfeld, Laura. "The Use of Blenderized Tube Feeding in Pediatric Patients: Evidence and Guidelines for Dietetic Practice (Chapel Hill, North

Carolina)." 5 Dec. 2013.

[434] Schoenfeld, Laura. "The Use of Blenderized Tube Feeding in Pediatric Patients: Evidence and Guidelines for Dietetic Practice (Chapel Hill, North Carolina)." 5 Dec. 2013.

[435] Meier, R. F., Reddy, B. R., and Soeters, P. B., editors. *The Importance of Nutrition as an Integral Part of Disease Management*. (New York: Karger, 2015), 1.

[436] Spruss, Astrid, and Ina Bergheim. "Dietary fructose and intestinal barrier: potential risk factor in the pathogenesis of nonalcoholic fatty liver disease," *The Journal of Nutritional Biochemistry* 20.9 (2009): 657-62.

[437] Gibson, PR, and SJ Shepherd. "Personal view: food for thought–western lifestyle and susceptibility to Crohn's disease. The FODMAP hypothesis," *Alimentary Pharmacology & Therapeutics* 21.12 (2005): 1399-409.

[438] Csáki, Katalin F. "Synthetic surfactant food additives can cause intestinal barrier dysfunction," *Medical Hypotheses* 76.5 (2011): 676-81.

[439] Rose, GA, WB Thomson, and RT Williams. "Corn oil in treatment of ischaemic heart disease," *British Medical Journal* 1.5449 (1965): 1531.

[440] Fernandez-Cornejo, Jorge, Seth Wechsler, Mike Livingston, Lorraine Mitchell. "Genetically Engineered Crops in the United States," *SSRN Electronic Journal* (2014)

[441] Akoh, Casimir C. and David B Min. *Food Lipids: Chemistry, Nutrition, and Biotechnology* (Boca Raton: CRC press, 2008).

[442] Severance, Emily G et al. "Subunit and whole molecule specificity of the anti-bovine casein immune response in recent onset psychosis and schizophrenia," *Schizophrenia Research* 118.1 (2010): 240-247.

[443] Severance, Emily G et al. "Seroreactive marker for inflammatory bowel disease and associations with antibodies to dietary proteins in bipolar disor-

der," *Bipolar Disorders* 16.3 (2014): 230-40.

444 Hollon, Justin et al. "Effect of gliadin on permeability of intestinal biopsy explants from celiac disease patients and patients with non-celiac gluten sensitivity," *Nutrients* 7.3 (2015): 1565-576.

445 Hadjivassiliou, Marios et al. "Gluten sensitivity: from gut to brain," *The Lancet Neurology* 9.3 (2010): 318-30.

446 Lê, Khanh-Tuoc et al. "Primary structure and expression of a naturally truncated human P2X ATP receptor subunit from brain and immune system," *FEBS letters* 418.1 (1997): 195-199.

447 Samaroo, Diana et al. "Novel immune response to gluten in individuals with schizophrenia," *Schizophrenia Research* 118.1 (2010): 248-255.

448 Lewis, Michael, Parviz Ghassemi, and Joseph Hibbeln. "Therapeutic use of omega-3 fatty acids in severe head trauma." *The American Journal of Emergency Medicine* 31.1 (2013): 273. e5-273. e8.

449 Wurtman, Richard J. et al. "Synaptic proteins and phospholipids are increased in gerbil brain by administering uridine plus docosahexaenoic acid orally," *Brain Research* 1088.1 (2006): 83-92.

450 Dafny, N. and NR Pellis. "Evidence that opiate addiction is in part an immune response: destruction of the immune system by irradiation-altered opiate withdrawal." *Neuropharmacology* 25.8 (1986): 815-18.

451 Kharrazian, Datis. *Why Isn't My Brain Working?*, 126-160.

452 Kharrazian, Datis. *Why Isn't My Brain Working?*, 128.

453 Davis, D. "Is gluten on the increase?" Wheat Belly (2013, February 15). Retrieved September 10, 2017, from http://www.wheatbellyblog.com/2013/02/is-gluten-on-the-increase/.

454 Morell, S. F. "Broth is Beautiful." The Weston A. Price Foundation, (2000,

January 1). Retrieved September 10, 2017, from https://www.westonaprice.org/health-topics/food-features/broth-is-beautiful/.

455 Toledo, Romeo T. "Postprocessing changes in aseptically packed beverages," *Journal of Agricultural and Food Chemistry* 34.3 (1986): 405-08.

456 Buchowski, MS et al. "Heating and the distribution of total and heme iron between meat and broth," *Journal of Food Science* 53.1 (1988): 43-45.

457 Wahls, Terry L. *The Wahls Protocol*, 323-25.

458 O'Bryan, Tom, *Autoimmune Fix*, 211-287.

459 Kharrazian, Datis. *Why Isn't My Brain Working?*, 95-100.

460 Mönnikes, H et al. "Role of stress in functional gastrointestinal disorders," *Digestive Diseases* 19.3 (2001): 201-11.

461 Bockelmann, B. A., & Bockelmann, I. L. "Aseptic packaging of liquid food products: a literature review," *Journal of Agricultural and Food Chemistry*, 34(3) (1986): 384-92. doi:10.1021/jf00069a001.

INDEX

THANK YOU TO ALLIES

Over the past few years, I have been honored to have the gracious support of many people, but three groups stand out as some of my strongest supporters. These groups do great work in neuro-rehabilitation and health. I wanted to recognize them here separately for their influence on my own recovery. My journey would not have been the same without their support and friendship. My deepest thanks goes out to each of them for being such great allies in my mission!

REVIVE TREATMENT CENTERS

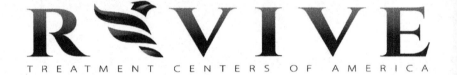

Revive Treatment Centers is a multidisciplinary clinic that focuses on post-acute care and neuro-rehabilitation for patients with concussions, TBI, stroke, autoimmunity, developmental delays, and neurodegenerative diseases.

They strive to provide tools that their patients can use to live better and love life more. By utilizing cutting-edge diagnostic equipment and procedures, they find the underlying cause of their patients' symptoms and conceive innovative treatment plans to best address individual needs. By coupling therapies to further drive neuro integration, their multimodal approach allows the activation of multiple pathways in the brain.

NORA
Neuro-Optometric Rehabilitation Association

The Neuro-Optometric Rehabilitation Association, International, (NORA) is a group of committed individuals from various disciplines whose focus is on advancing the art and science of rehabilitation for the neurologically challenged patient. NORA strives to make Neuro-Optometry a part of every multidisciplinary team which treats individuals who suffer a traumatic brain injury. They facilitate the communication and understanding of the paradigms of care within each discipline by bringing awareness and understanding of the need and importance of Neuro-Optometric rehabilitation services in serving physically and cognitively disabled persons.

PALEO f(x)™

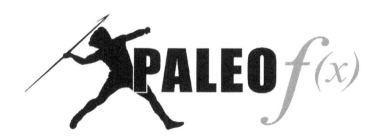

Paleo f(x)™ is an organization dedicated to three interrelated goals:
(1) To create the world's best holistic health and wellness event.
(2) To inspire and empower individuals everywhere to find optimal health and to flourish.
(3) To create a forum where ancestral health ideas can be turned into real world practices that improve human wellbeing.
Paleo f(x)™ is a forum where the theory of Ancestral Health turns into the practices that allow great health to flourish.

Made in the USA
Monee, IL
23 September 2020